A FAT LOT OF
GOOD

Dr Peter Brukner OAM is a world-renowned Australian sports medicine clinician and researcher. Until recently the team doctor for the Australian cricket team, he has held similar positions at Liverpool FC, Melbourne and Collingwood AFL clubs, the Socceroos and with the national Olympic athletics team.

A professor of sports medicine at La Trobe University, Peter is also the author of several books, including *Clinical Sports Medicine* and *Food for Sport*, and a founder of the SugarByHalf public health campaign. He lectures on health all over the world and appears regularly in the media, including Fox Footy TV, SEN Radio, ABC Radio and *The Age*.

www.fatlotofgood.com.au

A FAT LOT OF
GOOD

DR PETER BRUKNER OAM

All author proceeds donated to SugarByHalf.

PENGUIN LIFE
UK | USA | Canada | Ireland | Australia
India | New Zealand | South Africa | China

Penguin Books is part of the Penguin Random House group of companies whose addresses can be found at global.penguinrandomhouse.com.

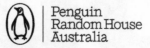

Penguin
Random House
Australia

First published by Penguin Random House Australia Pty Ltd 2018

10 9 8 7 6 5 4 3 2 1

Text copyright © Peter Brukner 2018
Recipes copyright © Penguin Random House Australia Pty Ltd 2018

The moral right of the author has been asserted.

Cover design by Louisa Maggio © Penguin Random House Australia Pty Ltd
Cover photographs by: StudioPhotoDFlorez/Shutterstock (avocado and broccoli); xpixel/Shutterstock (chocolate); AndriyShevchuk/Shutterstock (berries); bigacis/Shutterstock (butter); digieye/Shutterstock (nuts); Alabass27/Shutterstock (eggs); Plateresca/Shutterstock (salmon); vikif/Getty (olive oil).
Recipes by Chrissy Freer
Typeset in Berkeley by Midland Typesetters, Australia
Printed and bound in Australia by Griffin Press, an accredited ISO AS/NZS 14001 Environmental Management Systems printer.

A catalogue record for this book is available from the National Library of Australia

ISBN 978 0 14378 773 0

penguin.com.au

MIX
Paper from responsible sources
FSC® C009448

Contents

Foreword

Shane Watson
Australian cricketer

I have had the absolute pleasure of knowing Dr Peter Brukner personally from the day when he came on his first tour with the Australian Cricket Team in Dubai in 2012. Of course, I'd already heard about the famous Dr Brukner from my days studying anatomy and physiology at university, where we were using the textbook *Brukner & Khan's Clinical Sports Medicine* as our bible, to his high-profile work with the Olympic teams, the Socceroos and especially Liverpool in the English Premier League. So I certainly knew how privileged we were at the Australian Cricket Team to have someone of his calibre on tour with us to look after and guide us.

Doc Brukner (as I call him) and I spent a lot of time together on tour – especially our almost daily dry needling sessions, which he's a master at! – so I had the opportunity to get to know him extremely well. The thing that stands out to me the most about Doc is how much of a realist he is in an industry in which people get seriously caught up in all of the propaganda and the supposed truths that sweep up entire generations.

The big catalyst for my own low-carb, healthy-fat journey was on Australia's infamous tour of India in 2013, where Doc started to open my eyes up to another world of health principles that was so different to anything that I had previously studied, heard about or witnessed. Noticing that Doc had trimmed down quite a bit, I was very interested to find out the techniques he'd used to attain his svelte new figure – and so started my education about a world that I had thought I knew pretty well. As elite cricketers we were always told: load up on carbohydrates before a big game, and eat low-fat to keep your skin folds (or body fat percentage) at an optimal range. So I'd do a cycle of 'carbo-loading' before a day's play to ensure that I had plenty of energy in case I had a big day of batting and bowling. But in reality, if the day didn't work out to plan – as it often didn't – I ended up with all of this carbohydrate to store, which made keeping my skin folds at the optimal level a constant challenge. Now I can see that that approach just doesn't make sense.

Doc was very generous in sharing his tips from his personal experience, and thanks to his recommendations I also started to read some life-changing books: *Why We Get Fat and What to Do About It* by Gary Taubes, *The Real Meal Revolution* by Tim Noakes and *Salt, Sugar, Fat* by Michael Moss. They started me on a fascinating journey of self-education, explaining in shocking detail the misleading propaganda and cover-up of facts in the US in the 1960s, and giving me a new-found understanding of why I had a family history of type 2 diabetes. It also brought much-needed logic to my inexplicable battle to maintain my weight and skin folds even while devotedly following the dietary advice I'd been given as an athlete.

Doc and I would chat for hours about all of the various issues that surround people's health, good or bad, and how so much of this could have been – and still can be – prevented by providing everyone with very simple and, most importantly, accurate information that they can apply to their own lives. We have the right to know how simple it is to prevent the many diseases that cripple our society, and yet we're still being fed information that's incorrect, or from hidden sources, or subject to huge conflicts of interest centred around money and power instead of the needs of society and future generations.

That's why *A Fat Lot of Good* is so brilliant. You will never have to read any other book on this topic: it brings together all of the information that you could need to know about the myths and mistruths that have led us away from good health, and the practical steps we can all take to set us back on the right path for life. I have no doubt that you will enjoy reading it as much as I did and that this new understanding will be as life-changing for you as it has been for me.

Introduction

I'm Peter Brukner, a 65-year-old sport and exercise medicine physician, academic and author. I've spent the past 35 years looking after the injuries and illnesses of athletes, from recreational to elite, at the Olympic Park Sports Medicine Centre in Melbourne, which I founded in 1987.

I'm the co-author of the most widely read sports medicine textbook in the world, *Brukner & Khan's Clinical Sports Medicine*, and I've been instrumental in establishing sports medicine as a recognised medical specialty in Australia through the Australasian College of Sports Physicians, for which I was a founding member and have served two terms as president.

I have also been fortunate enough to be the team doctor for Melbourne and Collingwood AFL clubs; our national swimming, hockey, athletics, soccer and cricket teams; Liverpool in the English Premier League; the Australian Atlanta (1996) and Sydney (2000) Olympic teams; and numerous Commonwealth Games and World Championships teams.

So why would I give all that up? After all, as everyone tells me, it's the best job in the world.

Like most doctors, I was trained to believe that drugs and/or surgery are the answers to all medical problems. I was not particularly interested in preventive medicine, although I'd always had an interest in sports nutrition. In fact, I co-authored the first Australian book on sports nutrition, *Food for Sport*. But after that I gradually lost interest in that area of medicine. Like many members of the medical profession, I tended to be dismissive of any 'alternative' diets or lifestyle changes.

But all that changed a few years ago when my own increasing weight and health issues were not being resolved by the standard medical and dietetic practice. I was the doctor who became the patient, the person with a problem to resolve, or else suffer the consequences.

This led me to a journey of discovery, a realisation that turned a lot of the medical 'truth' I'd taken for granted on its head, and now I want to spend the rest of my medical career trying to change the way we live so we can lead longer, healthier lives. So I've written this book to share all the information that, if I were your doctor, I would want you to know.

We're all different. We have different genes and we've grown up in different environments, so it seems logical that we all have different requirements for a healthy, happy life. We each need a different diet, and different amounts of exercise, sleep, sun and so on.

Given these differences, my aim in this book is not to tell you how to run your life – that's your decision. I'm not going to tell you exactly what to eat for each meal. I'm not going to tell you how much exercise to do today or tomorrow. What I *am* going to do is give you the information you need, in as simple a way as possible, based on scientific evidence, to live a longer and – more importantly – healthier and more enjoyable life.

After my personal epiphany six years ago, I've spent the vast majority of my time reading everything I can on health, and in particular diet and exercise. New scientific research is being published all the time, most of it inaccessible to the members of the public who could stand to benefit most from its findings.

As a typical conservative medical doctor I thought I knew how to live, but on my journey of discovery I've come to realise that a large part of what I was taught and in turn have taught my patients, athletes, children and friends has been completely wrong. As a result, we have a horribly unhealthy society with high rates of obesity, type 2 diabetes, tooth decay and many other 'modern' illnesses that are now an enormous threat to our healthcare system and the life expectancy of future generations.

Our daily choices can take us a long way towards tackling these issues, which is why I feel compelled to share with you what I've learnt about the way to live a healthy life. This book will give you the latest information on all areas of health, and a set of principles you can use to build the lifestyle that's right for you.

It all starts with my own story, as the not-so-healthy doctor . . .

My Journey

It was 15 July 2012 – my 60th birthday – and time to take stock.

I considered myself pretty healthy, with no major medical issues to be concerned about. Five years earlier, I had nearly died from a blood clot to the lung (pulmonary embolus) and had to start taking a blood-thinning tablet, but I was on no other medications. I'd never smoked, didn't drink much alcohol, exercised regularly (a mix of walking and the gym) and followed what I believed to be a healthy diet, low in fat and high in carbohydrate. Like a lot of people, I loved my pasta, rice, potatoes and bread.

And yet despite following the dietary guidelines almost to the letter, I was overweight. In fact, according to the medical definition, I was bordering on obese. I'd probably put on 0.5 kilograms every year for the previous 30-odd years. As a result, by any reckoning, at 92 kilograms I was 10–15 kilograms over my ideal weight. My kids had started poking me in the belly and making cheeky comments about my ever-expanding abdomen.

Unfair, I thought. After all, I was doing 'all the right things'. But in the back of my mind I was also aware that my father had developed type 2 diabetes at 61 and that this horrible disease had led to significant complications that ultimately led to his death a couple of decades later. I didn't want to go down that track.

Soon after that birthday, I read something from my old friend and colleague Professor Tim Noakes, who is generally considered to be the pre-eminent sports scientist in the world. Tim had started advocating a low-carb diet without the usual restrictions on fat. He was on this diet himself with dramatic results, and was encouraging others, including athletes, to adopt it too. Tim is a lateral thinker who constantly challenges the orthodoxies of sports science. He wrote *Lore of Running*, a massive tome that's essential reading for any serious runner or sports scientist, and has fascinating thoughts on a whole range of topics (including cricket and Bradman's backlift!). So when Tim Noakes comes out and states categorically that everything we believe about diet, obesity and heart disease is wrong, we all need to sit up and take notice.

But surely, I thought, the medical, nutrition and sports science community could not have been so far off the mark for all these years in advocating a diet low in saturated fat (to prevent heart disease) and high in complex carbohydrates (to fuel exercise). And yet that's *exactly* what Noakes was saying. He even apologised for advocating a high-carb diet in *Lore of Running* – no doubt he will change that for the next edition.

Tim's conversion certainly got me thinking. I wanted to find out more.

Learning the truth

My first step was reading *Good Calories, Bad Calories*, by award-winning journalist Gary Taubes. This book critically examines the history of the diet debate and looks not only at the science of diet, obesity and heart disease, but also the politics, and how it came to be that governments as well as medical and scientific organisations came to recommend the low-fat, high-carbohydrate diet. For this book, Taubes spent four years analysing all the medical literature on the topic as well as speaking to all the major players in the field over the past 50 years. The result is quite amazing.

The wealth of positive evidence Taubes turned up shows that, contrary to what we've been led to believe, the traditional low-fat, low-calorie diet appears to be largely ineffectual, and in fact a diet low in carbohydrates aids weight loss and the reduction of various diseases. The key factor in controlling both blood sugar and blood fats (cholesterol and triglycerides), and ultimately hunger and weight, is insulin. But in spite of this evidence, as Taubes explains, the diet debate has been hijacked by the low-fat advocates – with subsequent disastrous consequences for our health. The epidemic of obesity is getting worse rather than better.

I was fascinated, but had contrasting emotions as I read the book. Although I was excited by the revelations and about how adopting this diet could have a dramatic positive effect on Western society, I felt depressed that my profession had largely ignored the science for 50 years. It was a confronting moment and the start of a new journey to get to the truth of the matter.

I began devouring books and scientific journal articles – anything I could get my hands on. I also became one of the nearly 7 million people to watch Robert Lustig's classic YouTube video *Sugar: The Bitter Truth*. The more I read, listened and watched, the more I became convinced that our current way of thinking about diet is wrong – but I was heartened to learn that there were lots of very insightful people out there who had challenged the dietary orthodoxies and were promoting a new way to eat. Welcome to the world of real food and low carb.

Putting it into practice

Armed with this new understanding, I decided it was time to do an experiment. Having done a little bit of clinical research over the years, I was fully aware that research involving one subject (n = 1) isn't scientifically valid. But given the '1' was me, I figured it was worth a shot. So I decided to drastically change the way I was eating. I eliminated nearly all carbohydrates from my diet and replaced them with healthy fats (see page XVI) while maintaining my protein intake.

Before starting on my new diet, I took myself off for some blood tests and had my blood glucose, insulin, blood fats and liver function tested. I also recorded my weight. My blood test results weren't too bad – or so I thought at the time – but in retrospect they showed that I was probably 'pre-diabetic' and on track to develop type 2 diabetes within a matter of years.

While my blood sugar was within normal limits, I had a number of other abnormalities that suggested I was heading down the same diabetic pathway as my father. My insulin level in particular was elevated, which was important given that insulin levels are now thought to be a more sensitive marker of impending diabetes than blood sugar levels. My blood fats were also slightly abnormal, with marginally elevated total cholesterol, slightly low HDL (often called 'good' cholesterol; see page 32) and markedly elevated triglyceride levels. (See page 308 for information on the significance of all these tests.)

The blood test also confirmed that I had a condition known as fatty liver or, more precisely, non-alcoholic fatty liver disease (NAFLD). This had been noted on previous blood tests over the years, but I'd tended to ignore these results, probably because I didn't really understand what they meant. I'll talk about fatty liver later in the book (page 8), but in brief it's a condition in which the liver becomes filled with deposits of fat. It was originally seen in alcoholic liver disease, but in recent years has started to appear commonly in non-alcoholics, probably due to excess sugar intake.

Now that I had my blood test it was time to start the diet, following the basic rules outlined below.

MY DIET RULES

My rules were pretty simple, if quite dramatic compared to my old eating habits. There would be no more sugar or junk food, but more importantly no more rice, pasta, potatoes, bread or cereal. There was no fruit juice, and the only fruits I would eat would be a few berries. Instead, I was going to have some of the things we'd been told for the past 30 years were bad for us: eggs and bacon, butter, cream, cheese, full-fat milk, grass-fed meat, cold-water fish (salmon and sardines), nuts and plenty of green vegetables. I wasn't counting calories, but was keeping a check on my total daily carbohydrate intake, aiming for a low intake of 30–50 grams, well down on my previous intake of more than 200 grams.

My results

The first thing I noticed was that my appetite decreased dramatically. Previously, after my breakfast of cereal, I would be ravenously hungry by 11 a.m., hanging out for an excuse to eat lunch. Now, after a breakfast of eggs, bacon and maybe some avocado, I didn't feel hungry at all, and most days didn't even eat lunch. If I did get a little hungry during the day, I'd have some nuts (usually almonds) or a piece of cheese.

Then dinner was meat or fish with lots of non-starchy vegetables – such as broccoli, green beans, zucchini, Brussels sprouts and cauliflower. Usually that was enough, but if I was still hungry I'd have a bowl of berries – strawberries, raspberries, blueberries – with full-fat cream. Drinks were plenty of water, tea or coffee (with a little full-fat milk) and the occasional glass of red wine.

I'd decided to weigh myself every Monday morning, and it was with great anticipation that I approached my first weigh-in. And I wasn't disappointed: I'd lost 1.8 kilograms in just seven days, which I though was a pretty good start. I had read that I might get flu-like symptoms in the first couple of weeks of eating this way, but I had no problems at all. I was also told that a lot of the initial weight loss would be fluid loss so not to get too carried away with the week 1 results. But I was encouraged by this early success and looked forward each week to the Monday-morning weigh-in.

And the success continued: I consistently lost 0.5–1 kilogram each week and was enjoying my food, feeling less hungry, sleeping better and feeling more energetic – I was no longer drowsy in the afternoons, for example.

Initially there was not much change in how I felt while exercising, but suddenly in week 6 I started to feel as if I could go forever. For the first couple of weeks I was a bit constipated, but once I started making my own 'muesli' mix of nuts and seeds that I ate with some full-fat Greek yoghurt each morning, everything started working normally again. In fact, the hardest thing was nothing physical – it was getting my head around the fact that all these fats I'd been told for 30 years were bad for me were suddenly apparently okay.

I stuck to this regime for 13 weeks, by which time I'd lost more than 12 kilograms. I was under 80 kilograms for the first time in God knows how long. In fact, my wife and others started telling me that I was looking too thin and should back off a bit. After those initial 13 weeks I did ease off a little, increasing my carb intake from the previous 30–50 grams a day to 50–80 grams a day. But overall I felt so good on the low-carb regime and it had shown such great results that it seemed like a no-brainer to keep going.

At the end of the 13 weeks I repeated my blood tests, with the following results.

My blood test results before the diet change, after my first 13 weeks and after five months

	Normal range (mmol/L)	My values (mmol/L)		
		October	December (13 weeks)	March (five months)
Total cholesterol	<5.0	5.4*	6.4*	6.1*
HDL cholesterol	>1.0	1.0*	1.1	1.15
LDL cholesterol	2.0–4.0	3.4	4.3*	4.4*
Cholesterol to HDL ratio	<5.0	5.4*	5.8*	5.3*
Triglycerides	<2.0	2.13*	2.16*	1.3
Triglyceride to HDL ratio	<1.5	2.13*	1.96*	1.13
Fasting blood glucose	3.5–6.0	5.5	5.3	5.9
Fasting insulin level	<10	11.23*	5.57	9.5
Liver function tests				
GGT	<50	56*	21	22
ALT	<40	65*	25	22

*Asterisk denotes a level outside the normal range

When I first looked at my week 13 results I was, to be honest, a bit disappointed. From my reading I'd concluded that the important results were my HDL cholesterol and my triglycerides as well as my blood insulin levels and liver function tests. After the first three months of my change in eating habits, my HDL and triglycerides hadn't changed much, but my blood insulin had gone down dramatically and my liver function tests, which had been abnormal for a number of years, had completely normalised – quite amazing.

After some further research, I suspected that my HDL and triglycerides may have remained high due to the breakdown of the fatty tissue I'd been carrying. Indeed, when I repeated the blood tests after five months, my HDL and triglycerides had both improved by significant amounts.

In summary, within just three months of removing carbohydrates from my diet I had:

- significantly reduced my appetite
- lost 12 kilograms
- lowered my triglycerides
- increased my HDL (good) cholesterol
- reduced my insulin levels

- resolved my fatty liver issues
- improved my exercise tolerance
- stopped snoring (and therefore had a happy wife!)
- stopped feeling sleepy every afternoon
- improved my energy levels.

Not a bad three months' work, I reckon!

There was one negative, though. I needed a new wardrobe. None of my clothes fitted. I went down two sizes in trousers and suddenly my jackets looked huge on me! But it was a small price to pay, I guess.

A whole new lifestyle

That was six years ago, and I've largely maintained that lifestyle ever since without difficulty. Once I got over the psychological barrier of 'fat is bad', I had no problems with the diet. I can still eat food that I enjoy: eggs with some combination of bacon, mushrooms, smoked salmon, or avocado, or my own 'muesli' of nuts and seeds with full-fat Greek yoghurt and berries for breakfast; cold meats, salads and cheese for lunch (if I have it at all); fish or meat for dinner with lots of vegies, followed by berries and cream for dessert. I drink water, green tea, coffee, bone broth and an occasional glass of red wine. My snacks have mainly been nuts (almonds) or cheese.

Over the past few years I've talked to a lot of people about the benefits of these changes. Many of the conversations were initiated by people commenting on my weight loss or how healthy I look. I've had friends, colleagues and many of the athletes I've worked with make changes that have made a huge difference to their lives. A number of the elite athletes I look after, including some of the Australian cricket team, have noted improvements in performance since changing their lifestyles.

For any way of eating to be sustainable, it needs to fit into a busy lifestyle – which for me, has meant spending the majority of my time on the road with the Australian cricket team – but I haven't found my low-carb, healthy-fat diet difficult to maintain while travelling. And while at first glance many of these foods appear to be quite expensive, I'll show you how it's easy to eat both healthily and cheaply with a few tricks up your sleeve.

Given the dramatic improvements in health markers that I've enjoyed, but most importantly the way I feel, you can understand why I've followed this lifestyle ever since and am now advocating it for you.

But first, let's do a check-up on the Australian population to see what kind of shape we're in . . .

PART I

The State of the Nation

Let's start by looking at our current state of health.

Where We're At

We are getting fatter and sicker.

Do you want the good news or the bad news?

Let's start with the good news.

The good news: we're living longer

Life expectancy among Australian men and women has slowly increased from around 50 years at the end of the 19th century to today's levels of 80-plus.[1]

The rate of increase is slowing down, however, and it's possible that sometime in the near future, life expectancy will start to decline. In the United States, a number of experts are suggesting that this generation of Americans will be the first to have a shorter life expectancy than the previous generation, the reasons for which will become obvious as you read this book.[2] It's likely that Australia will be in the same situation sooner rather than later.

OK, that's all of the good news . . .

The bad news

We might be set to enjoy increased quantity of life, but what about its quality? It's all very well to aspire to live longer, but if those extra years are marred by illness that prevents you enjoying the extra time with loved ones and doing the things you love, they can feel like more of a burden than a gift.

Let's have another look at those life expectancy figures. In 2012, a newborn boy in Australia could expect to live for 62.4 years without disability and another 17.5 years with some form of disability, including 5.6 years with severe or profound core activity limitation.[3] Girls born in 2012 could expect to live 64.5 years without disability and 19.8 years with some form of disability, including 7.8 years with severe or profound core activity limitation. What I'm interested in is how, through the health choices we make, we can extend those years without disability and reduce the years with disability – so that a bigger proportion of our lives can be enjoyed without impediment.

3

The six modern epidemics

In the past, we've had epidemics of flu, smallpox, cholera and Ebola, all infectious diseases that have been largely wiped out with the tools of modern medicine – vaccines and antibiotics. Unfortunately, we've replaced them with modern epidemics, not caused by nasty bacteria or viruses, but by the changes we've made to our lifestyles.

These modern epidemics are:

1   obesity
2   type 2 diabetes
3   fatty liver disease
4   tooth decay
5   cardiovascular disease
6   other chronic diseases (such as dementia, cancer, arthritis and auto-immune conditions).

Modern epidemic 1: Obesity

We're getting fatter – not just us here in Australia but in every Western country and even the developing world. In 2014 the WHO recognised obesity as a 'global epidemic'.

WHAT IS OBESITY?

The medical definitions of 'overweight' and 'obese' have been traditionally based on body mass index (BMI) results. You can calculate your BMI by dividing your weight in kilograms by the square of your height in metres. If you weigh 80 kilograms and are 1.8 metres tall, for example, then your BMI is:

$$80/1.8^2 = 80/3.24 = 24.7$$

BMI levels and weight classifications

Underweight	<18.5
Normal	18.5–24.9
Overweight	25.0–29.9
Obesity I	30.0–34.9
Obesity II	35.0–39.9
Extreme obesity III	>40.0

How fat are we?

In Australia, the proportion of the adult population who are overweight or obese has increased dramatically over recent decades. The Australian Bureau of Statistics' *National Health Survey* in 2014–15 estimated that 63.4 per cent of the population was overweight or obese – compared to 56.3 per cent in 1995. That means that more than 11 million adult Australians are fatter than the healthy average.

How Australian adults weigh in

Weight classification	Males	Females	All
Underweight	1%	2%	2%
Normal weight	28%	42%	35%
Overweight	42%	29%	36%
Obese	28%	27%	28%
Overweight & obese	71%	56%	63%

Source: Australian Bureau of Statistics, *National Health Survey: First Results, 2014–15*, 2015[4]

Nearly 5 million Australians are now classified as obese. Between 1995 and 2015, the proportion of obese adult Australians increased from 19 per cent to 28 per cent, of which an estimated 3 per cent are extremely obese, almost unheard of in 1995. We are right up there with the most obese countries in the world.

Proportion of obese people aged 15 and over, by selected OECD countries, 2015 or nearest year

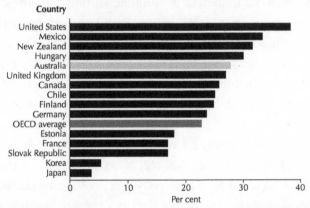

Source: Organisation for Economic Cooperation and Development (OECD), *Health at a glance 2017: OECD indicators*, 2017[5]

Men have more reason for concern: 71 per cent of adult men are now over-weight or obese compared to 56.3 per cent of women. Australia gets fatter as it gets older, too: of those aged 45 years and over, 79 per cent of men and 66 per cent of women are overweight or obese.

The trends among children and young people paint a hugely concerning picture for the future. More than a quarter of Australian children aged 5–14, and 37 per cent of young Australians aged 15–24, are overweight or obese. We know that obese children usually remain obese for all their adult lives. Australian girls rank in the worst third out of 33 OECD countries for overweight/obesity rates, and boys are in the middle third.

Obesity is particularly prevalent among those in the most dis-advantaged socioeconomic groups, Aboriginal and Torres Strait Islander peoples, and many people born overseas. Obesity is also more common in rural and remote areas compared to urban areas.

The cost of obesity

While obesity is associated with a large number of chronic diseases, and can have a major impact on quality of life and mental health, there's also a huge financial cost to the country. According to the *Fairfax–Lateral Economics Index of Australia's Wellbeing 2015* – which uses a range of indicators to measure our collective welfare – the cost to Australia of obesity has leapt by 84 per cent in the past decade to more than $130 billion a year, equivalent to about 8 per cent of the gross national product.[6]

In the decade between 2005 and 2015, the number of obese Australian adults grew from 3.2 million to 5.7 million. During the same period, the annual cost of obesity rose by $60 billion. Each 1 per cent rise in the obesity rate costs the nation $4.3 billion a year in wellbeing.

The increased healthcare costs associated with obesity are observable early in life, and recent research indicates that obese children between the ages of two and five incur healthcare costs 60 per cent higher than children of a healthy weight.[7]

Based on current trends, 2.7 billion adults worldwide will suffer from overweight and obesity by 2025. The cost of treating ill health caused by obesity around the world will top $1.2tn every year from 2025 according to *World Obesity*. They also predict that the rate of obesity in Australia will increase from the 2014 figure of 28 per cent to 34 per cent by 2025 if no action is taken.[8]

Why should we worry about obesity?

Obesity is a major risk factor for chronic and preventable conditions such as type 2 diabetes, heart disease, high blood pressure, stroke, musculo-skeletal disorders and depression. About 70 per cent of people who are obese have at least one established medical condition, resulting in medical costs about 30 per cent higher than people of the same age who are a healthy weight.[9] Many more have serious health conditions they're unaware of. It has been estimated, for example, that for every five known cases of type 2 diabetes there are four undiagnosed cases.

A recent Australian analysis of 12 studies involving 1.4 million people found those with a BMI over 30 have a 40 per cent higher risk of sudden death from heart attack than people of normal BMI.[10] The risk is highest among those who are obese from a young age. And most of those sudden deaths from heart attacks occurred in people with no other risk factors and seemingly normal hearts.

There is growing evidence that obesity is overtaking smoking as the major cause of preventable death in Australia.

Modern epidemic 2: Type 2 diabetes

Diabetes is a disease characterised by high levels of sugar in the blood. There are two types of diabetes: type 1 (or, as it used to be called, juvenile-onset diabetes) and type 2 diabetes (formerly known as mature-onset diabetes).

The diabetes problem

Based on data from 2014–15, an estimated 1.2 million Australians (5.1 per cent) have been diagnosed with diabetes, most of whom have type 2 diabetes.[11] It's thought that there may be up to half a million more Australians with undiagnosed type 2 diabetes.

Diabetes is more common in men (6 per cent) than women (4 per cent), and its prevalence increases with age to about 16 per cent for those aged 65–74. More than two thirds of people with diabetes also have cardiovascular disease and/or chronic kidney disease.

Every day in Australia, 280 people develop diabetes.
That's one person every five minutes.[12]

In 2013, diabetes contributed to 10 per cent of all deaths in Australia (15 100 deaths) – although in most of these (71 per cent), it was recorded as an associated, rather than the underlying, cause of death.

Diabetes costs Australia an estimated $14.6 billion each year.

Why should we worry about diabetes?

Diabetes is a problem because it brings with it many health complications. Diabetics have higher risk of:

- cardiovascular disease – angina, heart attacks, strokes
- nerve damage – numbness, loss of feeling
- foot damage – ulcers, amputations
- eye damage – blindness
- kidney disease – kidney failure
- dementia and Alzheimer's disease – which has been described as 'type 3 diabetes'
- skin infections – bacterial, fungal.

The statistics linking diabetes with heart disease, for example, are dramatic: 68 per cent of diabetics aged 65 or older will die of heart disease, and another 16 per cent will die of stroke.[13] Adults with diabetes are two to four times more likely to die from heart disease than those without.

Modern epidemic 3: Fatty liver

Many of you will have heard of, or even tried, foie gras – the French term for fatty liver used to describe a delicacy made from duck or goose liver. It's created by overfeeding the ducks or geese, a controversial practice that many people have tried to ban.

For decades, doctors have recognised fat build-up in the liver as a result of excess alcohol intake, a condition known as alcoholic fatty liver. In recent years, however, fatty liver has been increasingly observed in those with no history of excessive alcohol intake. We used to think that those with fatty liver were just denying their drinking habits, but we now understand that just as ducks and geese can develop a fatty liver by overfeeding, so can humans. This is known formally as non-alcoholic fatty liver disease (NAFLD), and is a relatively unknown but very important health condition.

About one third of all adults in the Western world are thought to have fatty liver, which would make it just about the most common disease there is. An estimated 5.5 million Australians, including 40 per cent of all adults aged 50 years and over, are thought to have fatty deposits in their liver.[14] Even children are now being diagnosed with fatty liver.

And yet most of these people are blissfully unaware of their problem.

Why should we worry about fatty liver?

Fatty liver is associated with a number of major health issues, including insulin resistance and cardiovascular disease, and is thought to be a step on the way to type 2 diabetes. Fatty liver can also lead to cirrhosis of the liver and ultimately liver failure, requiring a liver transplant. The burden of disease resulting from liver diseases other than hepatitis and cancer (the majority of which is NAFLD) was estimated as AU$7.5 billion in 2012.[15]

Modern epidemic 4: Tooth decay

Tooth decay (dental caries) is caused by the action of acids, produced by bacteria, on the enamel surface.

Fifty years ago most cities in Australia switched to a fluoridated water supply with the aim of reducing tooth decay. For 20 years the rate of tooth decay declined, but in the past 20 years, tooth decay in children has been increasing.[16] Nearly half of Australian children now have tooth decay, and three in ten adult Australians also have untreated tooth decay.

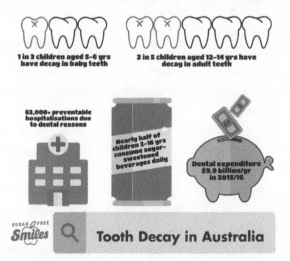

Reproduced with permission from www.sugarfreesmiles.com

Cavities, even in children who don't yet have their permanent teeth, can have serious and lasting complications, such as pain, abscesses, tooth loss, broken teeth, chewing problems and serious infection. Tooth decay in children is also a good predictor of tooth decay later in life. Each year in Australia, 63 000 children are hospitalised for preventable dental problems, contributing to our annual national dental bill of around $10 billion.

Modern epidemic 5: Cardiovascular disease

Cardiovascular disease (CVD) involves the heart and/or blood vessels, and includes coronary artery disease with its associated angina or heart attack (myocardial infarction), strokes and heart failure. The underlying problem for most of these CVD problems is hardening of the arteries (atherosclerosis), a build-up of fatty plaque in the walls of arteries that obstructs the blood flow. These plaques can rupture, causing a clot that blocks the artery.

CVD is the leading cause of death both globally and in Australia, where in 2012 it affected 22 per cent of the population. It's also our number-one cause of sickness.[17] In 2014–15, 23 per cent of Australian adults had high blood pressure, an increase from the 2011–12 figure of 21.5 per cent.[18]

While the death rate from CVD has decreased slightly over the past couple of decades, it's still a massive problem in our society. The reduction in mortality is probably largely due to reduced smoking and better emergency care of those who have heart attacks.

Modern epidemic 6: Other chronic diseases

I have already told you about the modern epidemics of obesity, T2D, fatty liver, tooth decay and cardiovascular disease. But there is another group of chronic diseases that are becoming more widespread – the final collective epidemic on our list.

In 2014–15, based on self-reported data from the National Health Survey, more than 50 per cent of Australians had at least one of eight chronic (long-term) diseases: arthritis, asthma, back pain and back problems, cancer, cardiovascular disease, lung disease, type 2 diabetes and mental health conditions.[19] Nearly a quarter of Australians – 23 per cent – have two or more of these chronic diseases. Chronic diseases cause 90 per cent of ill health, disability and death in Australia, and have a massive impact on the healthcare system.

Major long-term health conditions in Australia, 2014–15

Condition	Percentage of Australians affected
Mental and behavioural conditions	17.5
Arthritis	15.3
High blood pressure	11.3
Asthma	10.8
Heart disease	5.2
Type 2 diabetes	5.1
Osteoporosis	3.5
Cancer	1.6
Kidney disease	0.9

Source: Australian Bureau of Statistics, *National Health Survey: First Results, 2014–15*, 2015[20]

Dementia and Alzheimer's disease

Dementia is not one specific disease but rather a collection of symptoms caused by different disorders, of which Alzheimer's disease is the most common.

There are currently more than 400 000 Australians living with dementia, 55 per cent of them female and 45 per cent male.[21] About 244 people each day are joining the population with dementia. By 2025 the number of people with dementia is expected to increase to nearly 550 000.

Dementia is the single greatest cause of disability in Australians aged 65 or over, the third leading cause of disability burden overall, and the second leading cause of death of Australians. It places a huge burden not just on the individuals affected, but their families, friends and the community.

By 2025, some 255 800 home carers and 122 100 nursing home carers will be needed to cater for the expected increase in dementia. By 2025 the total cost of dementia is predicted to increase to AU$18.7 billion and by 2056 to more than $36.8 billion.

Cancer

Cancer is the leading burden of disease in Australia. It's estimated that approximately 140 000 Australians are diagnosed with cancer each year.[22] Three in ten Australian deaths are from cancer; one in four men and one in six women will die of cancer by the age of 85.

Mental illness

The *2007 National Survey of Mental Health and Wellbeing* estimated that 45 per cent of Australian adults will experience a mental disorder at some time in their life. It was also estimated that 20 per cent of the population had experienced a common mental disorder in the previous 12 months. Of these, anxiety disorders (such as social phobia) were the most common, afflicting 14 per cent of the population, followed by affective disorders such as depression at 6 per cent, and substance use disorders such as alcohol dependence at 5 per cent.[23]

Young Minds Matter, a national survey of the mental health and well-being of Australian children and adolescents, was released in 2015. Almost 14 per cent of children and adolescents aged four to 17 were assessed as having mental health disorders in the previous 12 months. Attention deficit hyperactivity disorder (ADHD) was the most common condition, affecting 7 per cent of children and adolescents, followed by anxiety disorders at almost 7 per cent, major depressive disorder at 3 per cent and conduct disorders at 2 per cent. Almost 30 per cent of those affected had two or more mental disorders at some time in the previous 12 months.[24]

Arthritis and other joint and muscle conditions

Arthritis is the major cause of disability and chronic pain in Australia, with 3.85 million Australians affected at a cost to our economy of more than $23.9 billion each year. By 2050, it's estimated that 7 million Australians will suffer from some form of arthritis. While there are about 100 types of arthritis, the three most significant – osteoarthritis, rheumatoid arthritis and gout – account for more than 95 per cent of cases in Australia.[25]

What do these six epidemics have in common?

These epidemics are global but are also affecting millions of Australians every day. As you'll see shortly, they all have three things in common:

1. They're a huge burden on our society.
2. We're not winning the battle to reduce their impact.
3. They're all related to the way we live, especially our diet.

> The World Health Organization (WHO) predicts that by 2020,
> two thirds of all disease worldwide will be the result
> of lifestyle choices.[26]

The WHO global burden of disease measures the impact of disease using the disability-adjusted life-year (DALY).[27] This time-based measure combines years of life lost due to premature death and years of life lost due to time lived in less than full health – and it shows that poor diet is the number one risk factor for disease, with tobacco the second most important. The Australian-specific figures show a similar story.[28]

Diet

The average Australian's diet has changed considerably in the past 50 years. During this time, the number of processed foods in supermarkets has increased dramatically. Whereas in the 1960s, 600–800 foods were typically available, there are now around 30 000 items in a standard supermarket, with many aisles devoted to highly processed foods (known as 'discretionary' foods) such as sweetened drinks, confectionery, savoury snacks, cakes, pastries, and sugary breakfast cereals and bars.

Processed foods are widely available in a huge variety of locations, such as petrol stations, sporting venues, convenience stores, vending machines, at the counters of retail stores, at leisure centres and in newsagents. You can even get them in my local post office! In some of these locations, processed foods are in the majority of items on offer, making it difficult for busy customers to find less processed and healthier options.

The average Australian adult obtains 36 per cent of their total daily energy requirements from 'discretionary' (junk) foods, only 49.8 per cent of adults eat the recommended two or more daily serves of fruit, and only 7 per cent eat the recommended five daily serves of vegetables.[29] A mere 5.1 per cent of adults and children meet both guidelines.[30]

We're now eating less red meat, full-fat dairy, fruit and vegetables, and more white meat, reduced-fat dairy, vegetable oils and processed foods with added sugars. The average Australian consumes about 16 teaspoons of added sugar every day, and teenagers have considerably more.[31]

We drink soft drinks, fruit drinks, sports drinks, energy drinks, flavoured coffees and teas – all containing added sugars.

We cook at home far less and eat more takeaway and junk food.

Exercise

Based on self-reported data from the 2014–15 National Health Survey, 56 per cent of Australians don't participate in sufficient physical activity, and this figure increases with age. Among 18–24 year olds, 45 per cent of men and 51 per cent of women met the recommendation of 30 minutes of moderate-intensity physical activity on at least five days each week. Of those aged 55–64, 54 per cent of men and 60 per cent of women were insufficiently active, while 75 per cent of those aged 65 and over were insufficiently active.[32]

The figures for children and adolescents are particularly worrying: only 29 per cent of children aged 5–11 and 8.2 per cent of adolescents aged 12–17 met the recommended 60 minutes of moderate to vigorous physical activity every day.

We will come back to the six epidemics and how we should tackle them a little later, but first I want to tell you how we got into this predicament and give you some of the tools to get us out of it.

PART II

How Did We Get It So Wrong?

As we have seen, we are getting fatter and sicker. Let's examine how it has all gone wrong. It's a fascinating (and somewhat depressing) story of money, power and politics.

Fat Versus Sugar

The theory that heart disease is caused by high dietary saturated fat and cholesterol has had devastating health consequences.

We've just seen that Australia and the world are in the midst of a rash of health epidemics. Seventy years ago, obesity was relatively rare, type 2 diabetes levels were low, dental cavities were uncommon, no one had ever heard of fatty liver disease, cardiovascular disease was almost unheard of, and people died from infectious diseases, not chronic disease.

Before the 1950s, few people had heart attacks, but during that decade the incidence of heart attacks started to increase. When US President Dwight Eisenhower suffered a heart attack in 1955, the public started to be concerned.

Two competing heart disease theories

At the time there were two competing theories as to the cause of narrowing or hardening of the coronary (i.e. around the heart) arteries, the medical term for which is atherosclerosis, which leads to a heart attack or myocardial infarction. One was that consumption of *saturated fat* was the major cause, the other was that *sugar* was the culprit.

In Britain, Professor John Yudkin was convinced that excess sugar intake was the cause of the heart disease epidemic. When he looked at the data on heart disease, he was struck by its correlation with the consumption of sugar, not fat. He carried out a series of laboratory experiments on animals and humans, and observed, as others had before him, that sugar is processed in the liver, where it turns to fat before entering the bloodstream.

He noted, too, that while humans have always been omnivorous, carbohydrates only became a major component of our diets 10000 years ago, with the advent of mass agriculture. Sugar – a pure carbohydrate, with all fibre and nutrition stripped out – has been part of Western diets for just 300 years; in evolutionary terms, it is as if we have, just this second, taken our first dose of it. Saturated fats, by contrast, are so intimately bound up with our evolution that they are abundantly present in breastmilk. To Yudkin's thinking, it seemed more likely that the recent innovation, rather than the prehistoric staple, was making us sick.

In 1972, the year his convincing book for the general public, *Pure, White and Deadly*, was published, Yudkin was unequivocal in his opinion of sugar: 'If only a small fraction of what we know about the effects of sugar were to be revealed in relation to any other material used as a food additive, that material would promptly be banned.'[1]

Meanwhile, on the other side of the Atlantic, American researcher Ancel Keys was promoting his diet–heart hypothesis on the basis of two studies: his Six Countries Study, which he claimed showed that consumption of fat was related to death from heart disease; and his Seven Countries Study, which narrowed the culprit down to saturated fat.

And the winner is . . . low-fat!

The story of how Keys' low-fat movement won out over Yudkin's low-sugar recommendation is a fascinating web of intrigue and corruption, documented thoroughly by Nina Teicholz in her excellent book *The Big Fat Surprise*.[2]

Keys first presented his data from the Six Countries Study at a symposium at Mount Sinai Hospital, New York, in January 1953 and it was published later that year in a paper entitled 'Atherosclerosis: a problem in newer public health'.[3] This was the first time Keys presented a graph (opposite, top) of the relationship between death from degenerative heart disease and fat calories as a percentage of total calories in the diet in men aged 45–49 and 55–59 in six countries: Australia, Canada, England and Wales, Italy, Japan and the United States. The six data points suggested a strong relationship between fat calories as a percentage of dietary intake and deaths from heart disease for men aged 55–59.

Keys concluded from this graph, 'Whether or not cholesterol, etc., are involved, it must be concluded that dietary fat somehow is associated with cardiac diseases mortality, at least in middle age.' Keys presented his graph of six countries with this explanation: 'So far it has been possible to get fully comparable dietary and vital statistics data from six countries.'

It turned out that data were actually available at that time for 22 countries, not six. The findings from the 22 countries are shown opposite (bottom),

Ancel Keys' Six Countries results

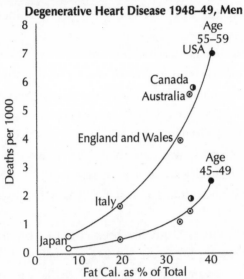

Source: Keys, A., J Mt Sinai Hosp NY, 1953[3]

Ancel Keys' data from 22 countries

Country
1. Australia
2. Austria
3. Canada
4. Ceylon
5. Chile
6. Denmark
7. Finland
8. France
9. German Fed. Rep.
10. Ireland
11. Israel
12. Italy
13. Japan
14. Mexico
15. Netherlands
16. New Zealand
17. Norway
18. Portugal
19. Sweden
20. Switzerland
21. United Kingdom
22. United States

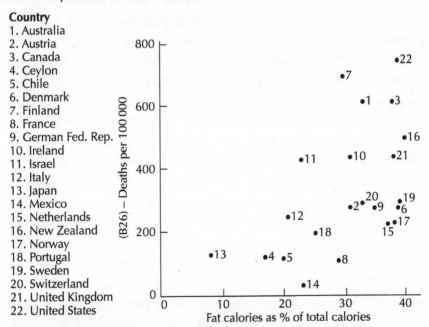

Source: Yerushalmy, J., Hilleboe, H.E., N Y State J Med, 1957[4]

and the researchers who uncovered it concluded: 'It is immediately obvious that the inclusion of all the countries greatly reduces the apparent association.'[4]

In 1956 Keys then embarked on his major study, the Seven Countries Study. Sixteen groups (cohorts) from seven countries were chosen: the United States (one cohort), Finland (two), the Netherlands (one), Italy (three), the former Yugoslavia (five), Greece (two) and Japan (two). Across these 16 cohorts, 12 770 men, aged 40–59, were studied (no women).

By the time the study was published in 1970, Keys no longer thought that *total* fat and heart disease were even associated.[5] The Seven Countries Study concluded that *saturated* fat specifically was the single dietary culprit in heart disease.

The Seven Countries Study has been criticised on many counts. On the basis of his previous Six Countries data, and falling victim to confirmation bias, Keys was aware which countries were likely to provide data that supported his hypothesis that fat was the key factor in the development of atherosclerosis. The study also had many methodological flaws, which should really have meant that its findings were dismissed.

Instead, despite a number of other studies with better methodology that did not show a similar relationship between saturated fat and heart disease, Keys' study became the orthodoxy. It was the key justification for the American Heart Association (AHA) to declare in 1961 that saturated fats were bad because they increased blood cholesterol, which blocked coronary arteries and caused heart attacks.[6]

The food industry then got in on the action. Vegetable oils started being manufactured in the millions of tons. Leading them all was Procter & Gamble, which began to aggressively market cottonseed oil – as well as making a sizeable donation to the AHA, an amount worth $20 million today.

After Keys, the next key player in this game was Harvard nutritionist Mark Hegsted, an ardent advocate of reducing fat intake as a means of tackling heart disease – although he recognised that this view was controversial. In 1977, the US government released its *Dietary Goals for the United States*, the result of a US Senate select committee examination of the American diet.[7] Although these guidelines were drafted by a researcher, Nick Mottern, he relied almost entirely on the advice of Hegsted. At the press conference announcing the first draft of the document, Hegsted stated: 'The question to be asked is not why should we change our diet but why not? . . . There are [no risks] that can be identified and important benefits can be expected.'[8]

Even the American Medical Association had genuine doubts, advising the Senate Select Committee: 'there is a potential for harmful effects for a radical long term dietary change as would occur through adoption of the proposed dietary goals'.[9] Despite this and other criticisms from many distinguished researchers, these concerns were brushed aside by the committee, which effectively endorsed the first draft and concluded that 'no physical or mental harm could result from the dietary guidelines recommended for the general public'.[10] Subsequently Hegsted was appointed head of the United States Department of Agriculture (USDA) Nutrition Center, which would be responsible for implementing the guidelines.

The role of the sugar industry

In 2016, documents were released that describe how industry sought to influence the scientific debate over the dietary causes of heart disease in the 1950s and 1960s. The sugar industry's major body, the Sugar Research Foundation (SRF), was especially concerned about emerging research indicating an association between the level of blood glucose and the incidence of heart disease. A 1965 editorial in the *New York Herald Tribune* concluded that the new research strengthened the case that sugar increased the risk of heart attacks.[11]

As a direct result of this editorial, the SRF established Project 226 with the intention of countering the threat to the sales of sugar. In July 1965, Mark Hegsted and his Harvard colleagues were generously commissioned by the SRF to produce a review of the existing evidence, with the aim of ending all doubt and showing that sugar was 'innocent'.[12]

The review, published in July–August 1967 in the *New England Journal of Medicine*, concluded: 'a lowering of the proportion of dietary saturated fatty acids, increasing the proportion of polyunsaturated acids and reducing the level of dietary cholesterol are the dietary changes most likely to be of benefit'.[13] In other words, saturated fat was denigrated while sugar did not even rate a mention. When the conclusions were reported by the media, saturated fat became public enemy number one. From this point on, the US dietary guidelines reflected the paper's conclusions.

Several biases coloured the results of this review. At the behest of the SRF, the most anti-sugar papers weren't included or considered, and the researchers played down links between sugar and heart disease while stressing those between heart disease and saturated fat. Most significantly, this review both directly and indirectly influenced public health policies for decades.

More recently still, further evidence has emerged of the role of the SRF.[14] In 1968 the SRF funded a research project on animals to shed light on the connection between sugar and heart health. But when the research pointed to a mechanism by which sugar might promote not only heart disease but also bladder cancer, the industry group ended the study and never published the results.

Hidden studies

Another tactic used by proponents of the diet–heart hypothesis was not to publish research findings that did not support their view – and that they therefore didn't want doctors and members of the public to know. The ongoing Framingham Heart Study, which began in 1948, has been recording the consumption of dietary fats and the development of heart disease among more than 5000 inhabitants of Framingham, Massachusetts. After the initial study period, the investigators found no correlation between fat intake, cholesterol and heart disease. These data, however, were never published.

As George Mann, one-time associate director of the Framingham Study later wrote: 'The diet/heart hypothesis has been repeatedly shown to be wrong, and yet, for complicated reasons of pride, profit and prejudice, the hypothesis continues to be exploited by scientists, fund-raising enterprises, food companies and even government agencies. The public is being deceived by the greatest health scam of the century.'[15]

Recently scientists have revisited data from two large unpublished studies from 1966–73. In the first of these, doctors intervened in the diets of a random selection of about 2500 people from the 9000 recruited for the Minnesota Coronary Experiment from mental institutions and nursing homes. For this group the saturated fats in their diet were replaced with polyunsaturated vegetable oil while a control group of similar size continued with their usual diet. Both groups continued for at least a year.

Recently, a group of investigators were able to obtain the raw data, which had never been published.[16] The autopsy reports from the 140 deaths that occurred during the study revealed that 42 per cent of the people in the polyunsaturated fat group had suffered a heart attack, compared with only 22 per cent in the control group. The amount of atherosclerosis in the coronary arteries was similar for both groups. While those eating polyunsaturated fat showed a 13 per cent reduction in blood cholesterol levels, the death rate in those over 65 years was 30 per cent higher. Would it surprise you to learn that the principal investigator in the Minnesota Coronary Experiment was Ancel Keys?

The second study, which took place between 1966 and 1973, is known as the Sydney Diet Heart Study. In this research, about 220 men aged 30–59 were instructed to reduce saturated fat intake and increase polyunsaturated fat intake. The men were supplied with safflower oil and safflower oil-based margarine (both rich in the omega-6 fat known as linoleic acid). A similar number of men got no dietary instruction and acted as controls.

In the results of this study, reported in 1978, the men who cut back on saturated fat and boosted their omega-6 intake were found to be at increased risk of *all-cause* death.[17] For some reason, the effects of the diet on risk of death specifically from cardiovascular disease (including heart disease) were not reported. When the researchers many years later went back to the old data to extract this information, they discovered that the men eating the 'heart-healthy' diet were at increased risk of dying from cardiovascular disease and heart disease (increases of 70 and 74 per cent respectively).[18] So, the very diet designed to reduce the risk of heart disease and fatal heart attack was found to have the opposite effect: it killed men, and specifically from heart disease.

Over the years, a nexus of industry, medical organisations and doctors supported by industry has promoted the diet–heart hypothesis. Industry has also continued to try and influence policy. In 2015, it was revealed that a group called the Global Energy Balance Network, which had repeatedly played down the link between soft drinks and obesity, was secretly founded and funded by Coca-Cola. It was forced to close after emails showed the extent of the relationship.[19]

So for reasons that had little to do with medical science but plenty to do with money, power and politics, Ancel Keys' diet–heart hypothesis has formed the basis of dietary policy for the past 30 years.

The diet–heart hypothesis: no scientific basis

The ideas promoted by the diet–heart hypothesis originated with animal studies and epidemiological studies back in the 1940s and 1950s. These seemed to suggest that dietary saturated fat and cholesterol could raise cholesterol levels in the blood. It was an easy sell: fatty food leads to fatty people, fatty arteries and ultimately strokes and heart attacks.

Dietary cholesterol and saturated fat
↓
Elevated serum cholesterol levels
↓
Atherosclerosis
(fat deposits on walls of arteries)
↓
Heart attacks and strokes

The only problem is that it was *not correct*. To understand exactly why, let's examine three assumptions of the diet–heart hypothesis and consider the evidence behind them:

- **Assumption 1: Eating foods containing cholesterol leads to high blood cholesterol levels**. High-quality scientific evidence indicates that, contrary to what the diet–heart hypothesis has led us to believe, dietary cholesterol has little to no impact on blood cholesterol levels.[20] The latest *American Dietary Guidelines* have actually acknowledged that fact. (For more on cholesterol, see page 321.)

- **Assumption 2: Eating foods containing saturated fats leads to high blood cholesterol levels**. Saturated fat does not have a major impact on cholesterol levels in most people. If it does, it causes elevation of both the 'good' HDL cholesterol and the 'bad' LDL cholesterol, cancelling each other out.[21]

- **Assumption 3: Dietary saturated fat increases the risk of heart disease**. A number of recent reviews analysing scientific publications have found no significant evidence indicating that dietary saturated fat increases the risk of heart disease or stroke.[22]

But if it's not cholesterol and saturated fat that cause heart disease, what does?

Experts in the area are becoming increasingly aware that the initiating factor in coronary heart disease is not high cholesterol, but rather chronic inflammation. This inflammation is aggravated by various lifestyle factors such as smoking; a diet high in sugar, vegetable oils and processed foods; inactivity; poor sleep; and stress (for more on inflammation, see page 56). The evidence now points to sugar and processed carbohydrates, rather than saturated fat, being the main dietary culprits.

This explains the steady increase in obesity, type 2 diabetes and other chronic diseases since the advent of the low-fat guidelines. Since we took the fat out of food and replaced it with carbohydrates, the results have been disastrous. For the past 30–40 years, the whole of the Western world has been part of a massive experiment founded on dodgy science – to see if reducing our intake of fat, specifically saturated fat, would reduce the level of these diseases. Instead the exact opposite has occurred: we have relentlessly increasing levels of obesity and type 2 diabetes in our communities.

What a disastrous failure!

The *Dietary Guidelines*

As we have seen, the wholehearted endorsement of the diet–heart hypothesis and the promotion of saturated fat as the dietary evil greatly influenced the development of the *Dietary Guidelines for the United States* in 1977, followed by Australia in 1982 and many other countries, especially in the English-speaking world.

The guidelines recommended a diet high in grains and low in fat, with vegetable oils taking the place of most animal fats. Despite concerns at the time from a number of researchers, the guidelines were adopted and soon became the orthodox view, remaining more or less unchanged to this day. Recently, researcher Zoë Harcombe re-examined the evidence available at the time and found there was no scientific basis for the recommendations to cut fat from the US diet in the first place.[23]

Thanks to the *Dietary Guidelines*:

1. **Intake of animal fats such as red meat, eggs and dairy was reduced**: Because of concerns about saturated fats, fatty meats were

discouraged and 'lean' meat promoted heavily. Eggs and dairy products, such as milk, butter, cream and cheese, were discouraged. Margarine was encouraged as a replacement for butter.

2. **'Low-fat' food products flooded the market**: The food industry responded to the dietary advice to reduce fat by producing a wide range of 'low-fat' foods. Because removing the fat from food also removed much of the flavour, they replaced the fat with added sugar or sugar-like products.

3. **Intake of ultra-processed foods increased**: Ultra-processed foods are products that contain several manufactured ingredients not generally used when cooking from scratch, including natural and artificial flavours or colours, sweeteners, preservatives and other additives. Some examples of ultra-processed foods include mass-produced soft drinks, sweet or savoury packaged snacks, packaged baked goods, chicken or fish nuggets and other reconstituted meat products, and instant noodles and soups. A recent study showed that more than half of all calories consumed in the United States come from 'ultra-processed' foods. I imagine the Australian figures would be similar.

4. **Use of vegetable oils increased**: Instead of saturated fats, the intake of polyunsaturated fats high in linoleic acid was encouraged as an alternative. Most prominently, the use of so-called vegetable oils (see box) increased dramatically. These included corn, sunflower, peanut, safflower, cottonseed, rapeseed, canola and soybean oils.

5. **Takeaway food grew more popular**: Fast foods – such as hamburgers, fish, chips and fried chicken – are cooked in vegetable oils because of their low cooking temperature and low cost.

During the course of the book I will be talking a lot about oils such as corn, sunflower, peanut, safflower, cottonseed, rapeseed, canola and soybean oils. These are clearly not from vegetables and strictly speaking we should call them 'seed oils', but as they are commonly referred to as 'vegetable oils', that is the term I use. Most of these oils are polyunsaturated (PUFA) oils – more on them later!

As the graphs below show, after the Second World War, consumption of sugar and vegetable (PUFA) oils increased, while animal fat consumption went down.

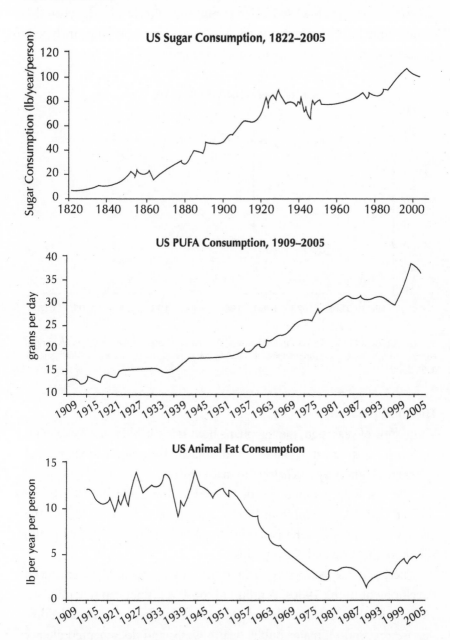

Source: Guyenet, S., Landen, J., *Whole Health Source,* wholehealthsource.blogspot.com

Looking back, it's now clear that the huge increases in the incidence of obesity and type 2 diabetes coincided with the dietary recommendations taking effect. The rates of obesity both here in Australia and in the United States (see graph below) started to climb from almost exactly when the dietary guidelines were introduced, while the start of the surge in Type 2 diabetes cases started a few years later. A coincidence? Sadly not.

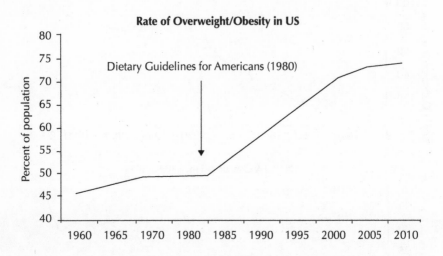

Rate of Overweight/Obesity in US

Dietary Guidelines for Americans (1980)

Source: National Center for Health Statistics (US), *Health, United States, 2008: With Special Feature on the Health of Young Adults*, Hyattsville (MD): National Center for Health Statistics (US), 2009

The food pyramid

Thousands of years ago, the Egyptians built remarkable feats of engineering known as the great pyramids. Unfortunately, the modern food pyramid has been significantly less helpful to mankind!

The first food pyramid was developed in Sweden in the 1970s. The original US food pyramid from 1992 was a graphical representation of the *Dietary Guidelines*, emphasising the bread, cereal, rice and pasta group over both the meat and dairy groups.

There's an interesting story behind the US food pyramid, which began development in the 1980s. A group of top-level American nutritionists, working for the USDA, combined research on nutrient recommendations, disease prevention, major public health issues and documented dietary deficiencies, and put the pyramid together in the eating guide known as

The original USDA food pyramid (1992)

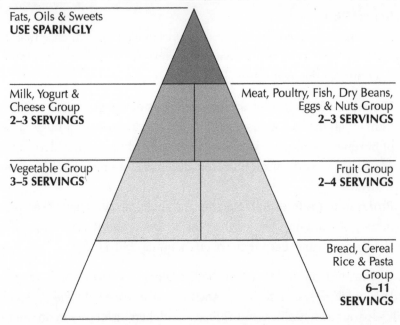

Fats, Oils & Sweets
USE SPARINGLY

Milk, Yogurt &
Cheese Group
2–3 SERVINGS

Meat, Poultry, Fish, Dry Beans,
Eggs & Nuts Group
2–3 SERVINGS

Vegetable Group
3–5 SERVINGS

Fruit Group
2–4 SERVINGS

Bread, Cereal
Rice & Pasta
Group
**6–11
SERVINGS**

Source: U.S. Department of Agriculture, U.S. Department Health and Human Services

the Food Guide Pyramid. However, when the guide came back from review by the Secretary of Agriculture, it had been radically altered: the servings of wheat and grain had been significantly increased; the recommendation for 5–9 daily servings of fresh fruits and vegetables had been changed to just 2–3 servings; and the guideline of 3–4 servings of wholegrain breads and cereals per day had been inflated to 6–11 servings. In fact, the peak of the pyramid – baked goods, sweets and other low-nutrient foods laden with fats and sugars, all to be eaten sparingly – had been moved down to be the base of the pyramid!

All these wholesale changes to the guide were designed to play to the interests of the food industry, such as the processed wheat and corn producers – despite the fact that doing so was in total disregard of the research basis by which the pyramid had been carefully developed in the first place.

So the food pyramid clearly needs some serious readjusting if it is to be as useful to modern society as the ancient pyramids were to the Egyptians! We'll get to the new food pyramid a little later on.

Why we haven't overhauled the *Dietary Guidelines*

Why does the saturated fat myth remain, despite all the evidence that it's false? Why won't the guidelines committee review the now overwhelming evidence and set the record straight?

1. **Vested financial interests**: There are considerable financial interests in maintaining the status quo. The food industry sells a huge range of beverages and processed foods, most of which have added sugar. The drug industry's most profitable drugs are the cholesterol-lowering statins.

2. **Professional reputation**: Doctors and dietitians who have been promoting the low-fat diet for the past 30 years find it very difficult to change their tune, despite the overwhelming evidence.

But we can't wait around for public bodies, global companies and even our outdated medical system to change their message. We need to take responsibility for our own health as individuals – and there's a lot we can do simply through our everyday food choices. That starts with challenging the diet myths and understanding the science – the *real* science – for ourselves.

JUNK FOOD IN AUSTRALIA

The LiveLighter website has an excellent review of the junk food industry in Australia. Its key messages are:

- Australians consume energy-dense, nutrient-poor junk foods so often as to cause concern.
- Large numbers of heavily marketed and promoted processed junk foods are sold throughout Australia.
- The junk food industry helps prevent policies and regulatory initiatives being implemented when they could impinge upon sales.
- Junk food is marketed to children with serious consequences. Legislation is necessary to address this as a political and ethical issue, and the ineffectiveness of the current self-regulatory and voluntary system.

- Despite the effects of their products on public health, the junk food industry is subsidised, directly and indirectly, by Australian governments.

POINTS TO REMEMBER
- The reasons the low-fat movement won out over the low-carb movement had more to do with ego, politics and money than it did with science and health.
- The diet–heart hypothesis falsely formed the basis of nutrition advice for three decades.
- As a result, the dietary guidelines and food pyramid were introduced without any solid evidence to support them.

Cholesterol: Bad Boy or Innocent Bystander?

*The cholesterol we eat has almost no effect on
blood cholesterol.*

For 30 years the medical profession has been obsessed with cholesterol, but as we've seen, cholesterol isn't really as bad as we've been led to believe.

What is cholesterol?

Cholesterol is a type of fat made by every cell in our body and is an essential component of the cell membranes surrounding each cell. Cholesterol plays an important role in the body, especially for cognitive function. Our brain makes up only 2 per cent of our body weight, but contains 25 per cent of the body's cholesterol. Many neurons are encased in fatty covers called myelin sheaths, and myelin is one-fifth cholesterol by weight. Cholesterol is also an essential precursor for vitamin D as well as all steroid hormones, including the adrenal hormones (adrenaline and cortisol) and the sex hormones (progesterone, oestrogens and testosterone).

Most of the cholesterol in our body is made by the body itself. Most importantly, *cholesterol ingested in food has very little effect on our total blood cholesterol*. This is because when our cholesterol intake from food increases, our body automatically decreases its own production, thus keeping cholesterol levels steady. All animal cells contain cholesterol, and for many years it was thought that intake of foods high in animal fat, such as eggs, shellfish and meat, led to elevated cholesterol levels in the body.

Even our old friend Ancel Keys admitted in 1997 that, 'There's no connection whatsoever between the cholesterol in food and cholesterol in the blood. And we've known that all along. Cholesterol in the diet doesn't matter at all unless you happen to be a chicken or a rabbit.'[1] The *American Dietary Guidelines* and the American Heart Association have since removed their advice to cut down on foods high in cholesterol.

HDL and LDL cholesterol – 'good' and 'bad' cholesterol

This is where it gets interesting (and controversial). A bit of background first.

First, all cholesterol is the same. HDL and LDL are not different types of cholesterol despite being labelled 'good' and 'bad' cholesterol respectively. Let me explain.

Cholesterol and triglycerides are not soluble in plasma, the liquid that carries our blood cells (i.e. they can't dissolve in water), and are therefore said to be hydrophobic (literally afraid of water). To be taken anywhere in our body, they need to be carried by a special protein-wrapped transport vessel called a lipoprotein. There are several types of lipoprotein, such as (in order of increasing density) chylomicrons, very low-density lipoprotein (VLDL), low-density lipoprotein (LDL) and high-density lipoprotein (HDL).

LDL particles are the major transporters of cholesterol around the body, taking it into cells where cholesterol is running low. HDL particles are thought to transport excess cholesterol back to the liver for disposal.

BLOOD CHOLESTEROL TESTS

When your doctor sends off your blood for a 'cholesterol' test, what you actually get is a series of measurements known as your 'lipid profile' (lipid is the scientific word for fat). Typically, these results are presented as below (with 'normal' levels in brackets):

- Total cholesterol (<5.0 mmol/L)
- LDL cholesterol (2.0–4.0 mmol/L)
- HDL cholesterol (>1.0 mmol/L)
- Triglycerides (<1.5 mmol/L)

This will be followed by at least one ratio, usually 'total cholesterol/ HDL cholesterol (<5)'.

Interpreting blood cholesterol tests

Initially the medical profession concentrated mainly on the total cholesterol result in blood tests, but over the past two decades the levels of LDL and HDL have been the main priority. LDL has been labelled 'bad cholesterol' and HDL 'good cholesterol'. Raised LDL levels have been associated with cardiovascular disease, and people with elevated LDL levels have been encouraged to commence cholesterol-lowering medication in the form of 'statins'.

As with most things in medicine, it turns out that it is not as simple as high LDL = bad news. There are two problems with that theory. The first is that the particles measured as LDL are not all the same and vary significantly in size from large, 'fluffy' particles, which are relatively harmless, to small, dense LDL particles, which are the ones associated with damage to the artery walls, leading to atherosclerosis and cardiovascular disease.

The second problem is that it is not the '*normal*' LDL particles that cause problems. They are only a problem when the LDL becomes 'oxidised', and it is the small dense particles that are more easily oxidised. Oxidation appears to be increased with ingestion of polyunsaturated fats, especially vegetable oils.

Unfortunately, the standard blood tests performed by most labs don't give sufficient information about the relative size and numbers of LDL particles, nor whether they're oxidised. It's possible to request a more detailed analysis of LDL particles, which will give the relative percentages of large and small LDL particles, but the blood triglyceride level is a good proxy measure of the level of small, dense (bad) LDL particles. If your serum triglyceride levels are elevated (>1.5 mmol/L), then it's likely that the majority of your LDL particles are small (and dangerous). Conversely, if your triglyceride levels are low, especially if they're <1.0 mmol/L, then it's likely that most of your LDL particles are the large, fluffy ones.

Triglyceride levels correlate well with cardiovascular disease, and I believe they offer a clearer indication of your risk of cardiovascular disease than your LDL level does. Triglyceride levels are usually elevated in overweight or obese people, and can be reduced by cutting down sugar and carbohydrate intake, and losing weight.

The important point to note about triglycerides in the blood is that they don't come directly from dietary fats, but are made in the liver from any *excess sugars* that have not been used for energy. The source of these excess sugars is any food containing carbohydrates, particularly refined sugar and white flour.

You may remember that my own triglyceride levels fell from an abnormally high level (2.3 mmol/L) to a 'normal' level (1.3 mmol/L) after three months of a low-sugar diet high in real foods and low in processed foods. My triglyceride level did not fall immediately after I lost weight (much to my initial disappointment), but had fallen three months later. I imagine that while I was in my weight-loss phase I was mobilising fat from my fat stores and thus my blood triglycerides remained high.

HDL is known as the 'good cholesterol' and elevated levels of HDL have been associated with reductions in the incidence of cardiovascular disease. HDL is thought to protect and repair LDL and fats from oxidative damage.

Instead of focusing on the total cholesterol or LDL cholesterol levels on your blood tests, I suggest looking closely at your triglyceride and HDL levels. I like calculating the triglyercide to HDL ratio. It won't appear on the report from the lab, but you can easily do the division yourself. For example, if my results were:

Triglycerides 1.3
HDL cholesterol 1.1

Then my triglyceride to HDL ratio would be 1.3/1.1 or 1.2. I like to aim for a ratio of less than 1.5, but certainly under 2 is desirable.

The triglyceride to HDL ratio has been shown to be a good predictor of the risk of heart attack. Those with low ratios have a very small risk of heart attack, while those with high ratios are at substantially higher risk.[2]

Cholesterol and heart disease

It's easy to see why the theory that cholesterol causes heart disease was attractive. When they examined the arteries of people with atherosclerosis, they found that areas called plaques where the hardening occurred were full of cholesterol. It was then an easy jump to say that excess cholesterol in the blood led to deposition of cholesterol in the artery wall, which led to narrowing of the vessel and plaque formation. And from there, that simply by reducing your cholesterol and fat intake, you would reduce the amount of cholesterol in your blood and therefore the deposition of cholesterol in the artery wall. All pretty simple and attractive as a theory: fatty food → fatty people → fatty arteries.

Only one slight problem. It wasn't true!

In his book *The Great Cholesterol Con*, British doctor Malcolm Kendrick examines the World Health Organization (WHO) data for the consumption of saturated fat in different countries and their rates of heart disease deaths.[3] He compares the heart disease figures for the seven countries with the lowest consumption of saturated fat with those of the seven countries with the highest consumption of saturated fat.

The results are emphatic. Every one of the seven countries with the lowest saturated fat consumption has significantly higher rates of heart disease than every one of the seven countries with the highest saturated fat consumption.

Kendrick then looks at heart disease rates in men from different European countries and compares them with cholesterol levels. He even includes data from Indigenous Australians, who have one of the world's highest heart disease rates.

Comparison between heart disease rates in men aged 35–74 and average cholesterol levels in 15 populations

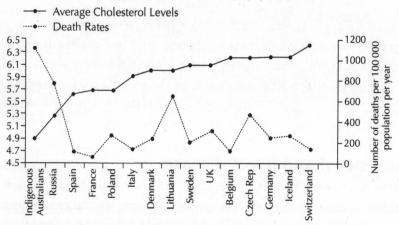

Source: Kendrick, M., *The Great Cholesterol Con*, 2007

As you can see from the graph, there is no link between heart disease and cholesterol levels.

Following on from Kendrick's analyses, Zoë Harcombe also used the full WHO data to examine the link between heart disease death and cholesterol levels in both men and women. Her work showed that higher cholesterol levels are associated with lower rates of death from cardiovascular disease, and lower cholesterol levels are associated with higher rates of death from cardiovascular disease.[4] In women, the relationship is stronger.

Harcombe then graphed the same cholesterol information against the total deaths from any cause – cancer, heart disease, diabetes, stroke. The even more dramatic results showed a significant association between higher cholesterol levels and lower death rates, and lower cholesterol levels and higher death rates, for men and even more so for women.

There's even some evidence that low cholesterol levels may in fact be dangerous, and high levels protective. Have a look at this graph with data from different countries showing that the higher the percentage of raised cholesterol in the female population, the fewer deaths from cardiovascular disease.[5]

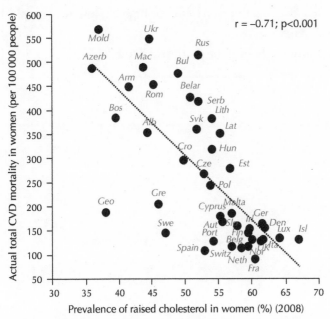

Source: Grasgruber, P., et al., Food Nutr Res, 2016[5]

If it's not cholesterol, what is it?

Blaming cholesterol for the plaque formation in atherosclerosis is a bit like blaming the firefighters for the fire – they're always there, but not necessarily the cause!

There's still considerable debate regarding the true sequence of events in the development of atherosclerosis, but there's increasing acceptance that inflammation is the key initiating event. A subsequent reaction from the body mobilising white blood cells to fight the inflammation creates a 'sticky' environment and the oxidised fats contained in the LDL particles are deposited there.

And the cause of that inflammation? Poor diet – excess sugars, processed foods and vegetable oils – lack of physical activity, stress, poor sleep and insulin resistance.

POINTS TO REMEMBER

- Cholesterol plays a vital role in the body, especially the brain.
- The most important blood measure is your triglyceride to HDL ratio.
- The evidence for a relationship between high cholesterol levels and heart disease is flimsy.
- Low cholesterol might even be detrimental to health.

Calories In, Calories Out

Our obsession with calories can finally end!

We've been obsessed with calories for years, but there's no need to count calories any more. Let me explain.

All calories are not the same

The first law of thermodynamics says that energy can't be created or destroyed. In the nutrition and diet industry, it's usually talked about in terms such as 'energy in must equal energy out' and is called the energy balance equation:

$$\text{Calories in} = \text{Calories out}$$

Or in other words:

$$\text{Weight gain (energy balance)} = \text{Energy in (food)} - \text{Energy out (exercise)}$$

We're told that the only way we can lose weight is to either consume less energy (reduce calories in) or burn more energy (increase calories out), but if only it was that simple.

Exercise burns calories so slowly, though, that very few people can find the time or maintain the willpower needed to affect energy balance significantly. The other problem is that exercising makes us hungrier.

Years of experience tells us that the calories in, calories out theory doesn't work. Yes, if we reduce our calorie intake we initially lose weight, but then our body wakes up to the change and starts using less energy. Our weight soon plateaus and then we regain the weight even if we maintain the reduced calories, because the body has adapted to less.

NUTRIENT DENSITY, NOT CALORIES

We're obsessed with calories. Diets are defined by the number of calories they include ('low-calorie diets'), foods are defined by the number of calories they have, and food manufacturers and even restaurants are encouraged, and in some cases forced, to tell us how many calories in a certain dish. But we don't eat calories, we eat nutrients.

Many foods contain empty calories, also known as discretionary calories – they provide the same energy as any other calorie but lack accompanying nutrients such as vitamins, minerals, antioxidants, amino acids and fibre.

Instead of calories, we should focus on the nutrient density of foods – in other words, the proportion of nutrients in a food relative to its energy content. Nutrient-dense foods contain the vitamins, minerals, antioxidants, amino acids and fibre missing from the empty-calorie foods.

Common empty-calorie and nutrient-dense foods

Empty-calorie foods	Nutrient-dense foods
Sugar	Eggs
Soft drinks	Meat – beef, lamb, pork, chicken
Fruit-flavoured drinks	Oily fish – salmon, sardines
White flour	Shellfish – oysters, prawns, mussels
Cakes, desserts	Liver and other organ meats
Biscuits, cookies, crisps	Avocado
Confectionery	Green vegetables – broccoli, spinach
Ice cream	Nuts – almonds, macadamias
Margarine	Dairy – full-fat
Vegetable oils	Mushrooms
Beer	Seaweed
Foods with added sugars	Cacao – 70+ per cent dark chocolate

While a small amount of empty-calorie food is fine, you should ensure that most of what you eat is full of nutrients.

Insulin and the hormonal theory of obesity

It is the *type* of food, not the number of calories that matters. Just consider 100 calories of ice cream and 100 calories of broccoli. No one could seriously contend that the two are equally nutritionally healthy.

When we eat sugar and refined carbohydrates they are broken down to glucose in the gut and the glucose is subsequently absorbed into the bloodstream. In response to this, the pancreas secretes the hormone insulin. Insulin works primarily to move the glucose out of the blood into the liver and muscles where it is stored as glycogen. Once the glycogen stores are full, insulin stores any excess glucose as fat. There is therefore a direct link between consumption of sugar and refined carbohydrates, and overweight and obesity.

Our weight and our ability to lose it is determined not by the *quantity* of food we consume, but its *quality*. The proportions of fat and carbohydrate are what matters. (For more on insulin, see page 49.)

POINTS TO REMEMBER

- All calories are not the same.
- Calories in, calories out doesn't work for weight loss.
- Insulin ensures that excess carbohydrate is stored as fat.

Salt: Too Much or Too Little?

Maybe we're targeting the wrong white crystal.

Along with saturated fat, salt has been demonised over the past 50 years. Too much salt is allegedly associated with raised blood pressure (hypertension), and health authorities recommend that we restrict our intake. And yet salt (in particular the sodium it contains) is essential for our health – *every cell* in our body needs sodium. This mineral has been part of the human diet for thousands of years, and has been vital for preserving food throughout this time, particularly before we had the luxury of refrigeration.

Salt and high blood pressure

We have already covered (and debunked) the diet–heart hypothesis. Well, here is another: the salt–blood pressure hypothesis, i.e. eating higher levels of salt leads to higher blood pressure. The theory is simple: excess salt intake causes the body to retain excess water, which leads to raised blood pressure. Reducing your salt intake will therefore lower your blood pressure. Sounds reasonable, right?

The history of how we got to this recommendation is remarkably similar to the fat story, which I guess is understandable given they both appeared around the same time, when nutrition science was so young it virtually did not exist.

The recommendation to eat less salt came from a series of studies by Lewis Dahl in the 1950s and 1970s.[1] In the first of these, he found an association between sodium intake and high blood pressure when he fed rats 500 grams of sodium per day. This amount is, however, almost 50 times the average intake, which makes the value of the study questionable. He followed up with several studies identifying correlations between populations with a high average salt intake and high blood pressure which, in a similar way to the Seven Countries Study on fat intake, were scientifically flawed.

42

The current guidelines on salt

To reduce blood pressure and lower the risk of heart disease, the Australian Heart Foundation recommends that 'adults eat less than 6 grams of salt (2400 milligrams of sodium) a day. This should be lower for children'. If you have high blood pressure, they recommend you reduce your salt intake to 4 grams (1600 milligrams of sodium) per day.[2]

Most international guidelines are similar. The USDA guidelines additionally recommend that people over the age of 50 reduce their intake to 1500 milligrams of sodium or lower.

For your reference, 2400 milligrams of sodium is roughly the equivalent of one teaspoon of salt per day. To convert grams of salt to milligrams of sodium, one gram of salt equals 400 milligrams of sodium. So 2400 milligrams of sodium is 6 grams of salt.

Most people in Western countries consume somewhere between 2500 and 5000 milligrams of sodium a day, well above the Heart Foundation recommendation. But most of this salt people are taking in comes not from what they shake over their dinner plates, but from ultra-processed food.

Is there evidence for these guidelines?

In summarising the vast amount of research into the effect of salt on health in general, and on high blood pressure specifically, we can make three points:

1. The lowest risk of death and cardiovascular events seems to occur with sodium intakes of between 3 grams per day and 6 grams per day (equivalent to 7.5–15 grams of salt). In a huge study involving over 100 000 individuals in 17 countries, an estimated sodium intake between 3 and 6 grams per day was associated with a lower risk of death and cardiovascular events than was either a higher or lower estimated level of intake.[3]
2. Increased salt intake does not appear to be associated with high blood pressure (hypertension) until the dosage of salt gets extremely high (greater than 9 grams per day).[4]
3. Reducing salt intake has a minimal effect on blood pressure in those with normal blood pressure and a moderate reduction in those with high blood pressure.[5]

The effect of reducing salt on blood pressure appears to depend on whether or not you are 'salt-sensitive'. Only about 20 per cent of people without high blood pressure are salt-sensitive, while the figure is 40–50 per cent for those with high blood pressure.[6]

More importantly, though, there is *no* good evidence that a reduced salt intake has any positive effect on heart attacks or strokes. There's even some evidence that low salt intake may worsen heart failure and type 2 diabetes.[7]

When salt intake is reduced, the body responds by trying to retain salt and water, so the kidneys excretes less salt, the arteries narrow due to the reduced blood volume, and the heart has to pump harder. Blood viscosity is increased, which increases the risk of blood clots that could lead to heart attack and stroke, as are blood triglyceride levels.[8]

In other words, it can actually have a negative effect on the cardio-vascular system.

Salt and insulin resistance

The other problem with a low salt intake is its effect on insulin resistance. A number of studies have shown increased insulin levels in those on low-salt diets.[9] This is a key indicator of insulin resistance, which plays a primary role in the development of chronic diseases such as type 2 diabetes. Insulin resistance is probably the single most important factor in our health, so it's really important to understand what it is, how it happens and what the consequences are – see the next section for more. Low-salt diets also increase the synthesis of fatty acids in the liver, which can contribute to the development of fatty liver (see page 261).

For all these reasons, too low a sodium intake can be just as dangerous as getting too much. As with all essential nutrients, the graph for disease risk and sodium intake is actually U-shaped: both low and high sodium intakes are associated with increased risk of cardiovascular disease and death from any cause.

Salt vs sugar

Many scientists now believe we've been targeting the wrong white crystal in our search for the cause of raised blood pressure.[10] There's increasing acknowledgement that sugar, not salt, is the key factor here.

One of the reasons for the confusion around salt and sugar is that both are present in high amounts in processed foods. When people cut down on processed foods (e.g. with the DASH diet), this seems to be associated with improvements in blood pressure, and this has been attributed to the reduction in sodium intake. But processed foods are full of sugar, and it seems quite likely that it's actually this sugar that causes the majority of the adverse effects.

Sodium vs potassium

Another factor that can have a significant impact on whether salt will harm or help your health is the ratio between sodium and potassium intake. Imbalance in this sodium–potassium ratio can lead to high blood pressure, and the easiest way to achieve this imbalance is by consuming a diet of processed foods, which are notoriously low in potassium and high in sodium.

According to one study, the people at greatest risk of cardiovascular disease were eating too much sodium and too little potassium.[11] The risk of dying of a heart attack was more than twice as high for those eating lots of salt and very little potassium as for those eating about equal amounts. Foods high in potassium include avocados, pumpkin, spinach, sweet potato, salmon and bananas.

People with an insufficient salt intake are also at increased risk of iodine deficiency.[12] Iodine is critical for our thyroid health, and iodine can be difficult to obtain from dietary sources.

How much salt should we eat?

The optimal daily sodium intake will differ from person to person, and depends on various lifestyle factors such as activity level and current health. As mentioned previously, the recommended salt intake is 'a maximum of' 2500 milligrams of sodium per day (about 6 grams salt or one teaspoon). While there is undoubtedly a subset of salt-sensitive people who would benefit from lowering their sodium intake – those with high blood pressure and a very high sodium intake (more than 6000 milligrams a day) – this is clearly too low for most people. A recent study published in the prestigious medical journal *The Lancet* concluded that regardless of whether people have high blood pressure, low sodium intake (<3000 milligrams/day) is associated with more heart attacks, strokes, and deaths compared to average intake.[13]

I would recommend somewhere between 3200 and 4800 milligrams of sodium a day, which equates to 8–12 grams of salt or 1¼–2 teaspoons of salt a day. Having said that, some people should definitely be at the upper end of that range and maybe even higher. Those needing more salt include those who:

- do endurance exercise in hot, humid conditions
- sweat a lot
- are pregnant or breastfeeding
- are taking diuretic medication
- have kidney disease or inflammatory bowel disease
- are on a low-carb diet.

People eating a real-food, low-carbohydrate or ketogenic diet definitely need to increase their sodium intake, especially in the first few weeks of their diet. Low-carb diets (and prolonged fasting) cause a reduction in total body sodium. Raised ketone levels and reduced insulin both contribute to this sodium loss. People on these diets should add salt to their foods at every opportunity.

When I first adopted my nutrient-dense, low-carb lifestyle, I started getting nocturnal leg cramps, which made me suspect that I was low in sodium. When I looked into my diet I realised that without processed foods there was no longer much salt in my diet. I now add salt to my foods whenever I can – sprinkled on my eggs, meat and vegetables, and added when cooking – and I try to eat salted foods such as nuts. I do have a couple of weird ones, too: I add salt to both my green tea and my bone broth! Since adding salt, I've had fewer problems with leg cramps and my blood pressure is still a healthy 110/70.

POINTS TO REMEMBER
- Salt is essential for every cell in the body.
- There's very little evidence that excessive salt intake causes high blood pressure.
- We should avoid both very high and very low salt intakes and aim for a daily intake of 1¼–2 teaspoons of salt.

PART III

The Real Causes

Now we've established that cholesterol, calories and salt are not as important as we have been led to believe, let's look at what is really important. In this next section I am going to discuss three factors that are inter-related and all really important to understand along our journey to better health:

1. *Insulin resistance*
2. *Inflammation*
3. *The gut microbiome*

Then I'll explain more about how carbohydrates, fats and protein all function and the ratios we really need of each.

Insulin Resistance

Eating too much carbohydrate leads to insulin resistance,
a gateway to disease.

You may have seen the title of this chapter and thought, 'Oh that looks a bit technical, I'll skip that bit.' Well don't. Why not?

Because insulin resistance is probably the single most important factor in our health and it is really important to understand what it is, how it happens and what the consequences are. Now, I'll admit it isn't the easiest of concepts to get your head around, but I'll do my best to keep it simple.

You have probably heard of insulin as the drug that type 1 diabetics have to inject a few times a day to keep their sugar levels under control. Those with type 1 diabetes certainly need insulin, as they don't produce any themselves – for reasons that are not yet completely understood, the pancreas of type 1 diabetics stops producing insulin.

Prior to the discovery of insulin by Banting and his colleagues in 1921, those with type 1 diabetes invariably died and doctors could do nothing to stop it. Insulin changed all that and is still the basis of treatment of this condition. But while insulin has been a saviour for those diabetics, it causes problems for the rest of us. Let me explain with a very quick and simple Biochemistry 101!

Insulin is a hormone secreted by the pancreas, which sits in the abdomen. When we eat a carbohydrate food, the carbohydrate is broken down into glucose in the gut and absorbed into the bloodstream. That's when insulin gets to work.

Its role is to move the glucose out of the blood and into the tissues, especially the brain and the muscles, where it can be stored as glycogen (the body's storage form for carbohydrate) for later use as a fuel. Once the storage capacity for glycogen in the liver and muscles is complete, insulin takes the excess glucose to the liver, where it is converted into fat. That fat will only be mobilised for fuel *when insulin levels drop*.

In a normal system, insulin and glucose levels drop after the glucose from a meal has been absorbed into the tissues, the body responds by feeling hungry and the brain tells us to eat again. This is why we feel much hungrier a few hours after a carbohydrate-dominated meal, especially one with a big sugar load, than after a meal of protein and fats.

When the diet is consistently high in carbohydrate, in the form of sugar or other carbs such as starches or grains, the level of insulin in the blood remains elevated. This both:

1. leads to storage of the excess carbohydrate as fat, and
2. prevents the breakdown of fat when we need fuel.

A third effect of long-term high blood insulin levels is that after a time, the body's tissues become *resistant* to its effects. Just as an alcoholic's body becomes tolerant to alcohol, so too do our bodies become tolerant to insulin.

It was traditionally thought that obesity was the main cause of type 2 diabetes, and there's certainly an association between the two, but the modern thinking is that insulin resistance is the cause of both obesity and type 2 diabetes.

Overweight		Obese
Insulin Sensitive	High CHO intake	Insulin Resistant
Hyperinsulinemia		Metabolic syndrome Type 2 diabetes Chronic diseases

The main cause of insulin resistance is a diet full of sugar and highly processed foods. The high glucose load from these foods leads to high insulin levels (hyperinsulinemia), eventually leading to insulin resistance. Other factors can also contribute to the development of insulin resistance, including poor sleep (see page 219) and lack of physical activity (see page 207).

ARE YOU INSULIN RESISTANT?

If you are obese, and have metabolic syndrome, type 2 diabetes or cardiovascular disease, you can be pretty certain that you're insulin resistant. If your waist is over 80 cm (female) or 94 cm (men) then you may be 'at risk'. If your waist is over 88 cm (women) and 102 cm (men) the risk is higher. Another way of considering this is that if your weight (kg) is more than half your height (cm) you are at risk and should have further tests.

The presence of insulin resistance can and should be confirmed by your doctor rather than by self-diagnosis. The main measurable sign of insulin resistance is constantly high insulin levels in the blood, for which the medical term is hyperinsulinemia. This can be measured directly with a blood test of your fasting blood insulin level. Blood insulin levels are not commonly tested, but they should be part of your regular blood work-up, so make sure you mention it to your GP. Your blood insulin level should be less than 9 mU/L.

A more exact way of detecting insulin resistance is to measure your insulin response to a glucose load (a precise dose of pure glucose), in a similar way to a glucose tolerance test (see the Toolkit at the end of the book).[1]

Another way of detecting insulin resistance is the homeostatic model assessment (HOMA) test, which is calculated with this formula:

HOMA insulin resistance test = blood glucose ×
serum insulin divided by 22.5

(Note that in the United States, where blood glucose and insulin levels are measured in different units, the division factor is 405.)

Levels should be below 3.

There are online calculators for this such as https://sasl.unibas.ch/11calculators-HOMA.php

Another indirect measurement that may be indicative of insulin resistance is your triglyceride to HDL cholesterol (TG:HDL) ratio, described in the cholesterol section (see page 32), which should be less than 1.5.

What being insulin resistant means

If you're insulin resistant, you're at risk of becoming obese (if you're not already), and developing a range of diseases, including metabolic syndrome, high blood pressure, type 2 diabetes, cardiovascular disease, cancer, neurological disease and, for women, polycystic ovary syndrome (PCOS).

Back in the 1990s, Gerald Reaven, who first described what is now known as *metabolic syndrome*, conducted an experiment with a group of 208 'apparently healthy', non-obese volunteers (98 men, 110 women), determined their level of insulin resistance and then divided them into three groups – low, medium and high insulin resistance.[2]

Doctors followed these people for an average of about 6 years and kept an eye out for high blood pressure, heart disease, stroke, type 2 diabetes and cancer. They found a total of 40 of these diseases in 37 of the volunteers, and all of the diseases occurred in those who had some degree of insulin resistance. Those with little to no insulin resistance had no disease, those in the middle had some disease, and those with the highest insulin resistance had the greatest number of diseases.

Insulin resistance and chronic disease

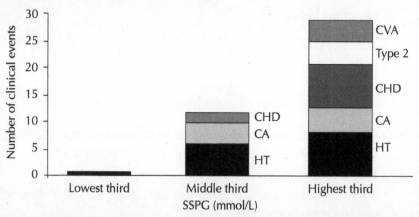

HT = hypertension (high blood pressure), CA = cancer, CHD = coronary heart disease, Type 2 = type 2 diabetes, CVA = cerebrovascular accident (stroke), SSPG = steady-state plasma glucose level (another measure of insulin resistance)

Source: Facchini, F.S., et al., *J Clin Endocrinol Metab*, 2001[2]

Two very interesting points come out of this study:

1. the close relationship between the degree of insulin resistance and the common medical conditions of Western society: high blood pressure, heart disease, stroke, type 2 diabetes and cancer, and
2. those involved in this experiment were all 'healthy, non-obese subjects' – and yet many were already insulin resistant, suggesting that many people have unrecognised insulin resistance and will go on to develop obesity and chronic diseases if they persist with their current lifestyle.

Insulin resistance has been shown to be a better predictor of cardiovascular disease than LDL cholesterol.[3]

> Insulin resistance is like an iceberg where most of the risk is submerged and out of sight.

Combating insulin resistance

Obese people often reference the fact that they know someone who eats the same as they do and does the same amount of exercise, but is skinny. This may be because the slimmer person is insulin sensitive, while the obese person is insulin resistant.

The good news is that you can reverse insulin resistance by addressing its causes, especially through the food you eat, your sleep and your exercise level. A real-food diet will reduce the glucose load, lower insulin levels and reduce insulin resistance, thereby decreasing the risk of complications such as type 2 diabetes and other chronic diseases.

Insulin resistance and carb intake

If you're clearly insulin sensitive and therefore able to metabolise carbs efficiently, then a moderate intake of carbs, perhaps 100–150 grams per day, is fine. I would still suggest severely restricting your intake of sugar and highly processed foods.

If, on the other hand, you're significantly insulin resistant, you need to severely limit your intake of all carbs. Again, depending on your degree of insulin resistance and your health aims (e.g. weight loss, control of blood sugars), you can adjust your carb intake.

Moderate your intake of carbs depending on your level of insulin resistance

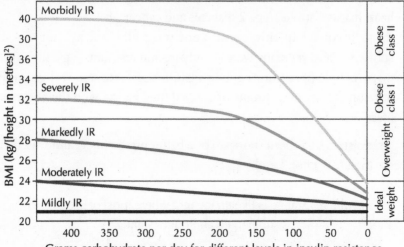

Graph showing relationship of amount of carbohydrates eaten each day to BMI in those with varying degrees of insulin resistance. The more insulin resistant one is, the greater the degree of obesity for a given carbohydrate intake. Those who are severely insulin resistant need to cut down their carbohydrate intake.

If you're already diabetic and/or obese and want to lose weight, then a very low-carb intake, probably less than 50 grams per day, is appropriate. You might even want to go as far as a ketogenic diet, which usually requires a carb intake of less than 30 grams per day (see page 179).

You might want to undertake a short period (e.g. three months) of severely restricted carb intake to get your diabetes and/or weight under control and then ease off. Unfortunately, there are no rules, and it requires a bit of trial and error with the help of your doctor, but you'll soon work out how many carbs you should have in order to achieve your health goals.

Constant eating

Eating patterns have changed quite markedly over the past 50 years. When I was growing up in the 1960s there were limited snack foods available and it was very much three meals a day. My mother was always saying to me, 'Don't snack, it will spoil your dinner.' Nowadays there's a tendency to snack constantly, and it's not unusual for adults and children to have three full meals and two or three snacks a day. This has a significant effect on our insulin levels, as the diagrams below show.

Insulin levels in the 1960s: three meals a day, no snacks

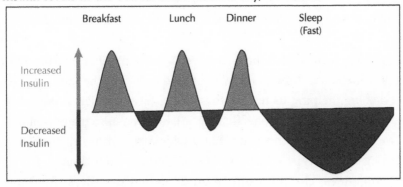

Insulin levels nowadays: constant snacking

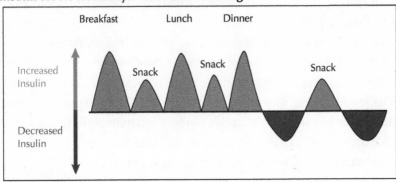

Source: Weightology[4]

POINTS TO REMEMBER
- The hormone insulin plays a vital role in the development of obesity and chronic disease.
- After long-term exposure to high levels of insulin from a high-sugar diet, the body's tissues become resistant to the effects of insulin.
- If you're insulin resistant you're at risk of developing type 2 diabetes and other chronic diseases.

Inflammation

We're realising that inflammation is the root cause of chronic disease.

Inflammation is the body's short-term response to injury or infection, and is largely mediated through the white blood cells. For the most part, it's a good thing, helping us resolve these short-term problems. When the inflammation becomes chronic (long term), however, it's a major problem.

We're increasingly realising that a wide array of health problems, including obesity, type 2 diabetes, atherosclerosis, heart disease, stroke, some migraines, chronic pain, attention deficit disorders (ADD and ADHD), asthma, thyroid issues, dental problems, osteoporosis and cancer are all rooted in chronic inflammation, which must be properly addressed if we wish to be healed.

The standard medical treatment for chronic inflammation is anti-inflammatory medications such as non-steroidal anti-inflammatories (NSAIDs) like aspirin and ibuprofen, more powerful corticosteroids such as prednisolone, and immune modulators like etanercept (Enbrel). A much more efficient way to tackle chronic inflammation, though, is to look for the sources of that inflammation and eliminate them.

The main contributors to chronic inflammation are:

- a diet high in sugar, processed foods and the inflammatory fats found in vegetable oils
- lack of exercise
- excessive stress
- inadequate sleep
- food allergies and sensitivities – to dairy, gluten and FODMAPs (see page 169)
- chronic infections – viral, bacterial, fungal (yeasts) or parasitic
- environmental toxins.

Altering the diet to reduce substances that promote inflammation has been shown to be an effective form of treatment.[1]

The main dietary inflammation provokers are:

- sugar and sugar equivalents
- trans fats (in partially hydrogenated oils)
- vegetable oils
- refined carbohydrates
- excessive alcohol
- processed meats.

The ideal anti-inflammatory diet is one that avoids those foods and is full of the healthy, real, unprocessed foods that I will describe later in this book.

MEASURING INFLAMMATION

A number of blood markers are raised in people with acute and chronic inflammation. The most commonly used marker is C-reactive protein (CRP) level. Usually, there's little if any CRP in the blood so any level above 3 mg/L is considered to indicate inflammation. CRP levels can be lowered by addressing the possible causes of the inflammation. More recently, a newer, more sensitive CRP test, high-sensitivity CRP (hs-CRP), has been found useful in identifying those at increased risk of CVD (see What Blood Tests Should I Have?, page 308).

Inflammation and insulin resistance

A recent study from Korea showed a correlation between measures of insulin resistance (high blood insulin, high triglyceride to HDL ratio) and CRP, the most commonly used measure of inflammation.[2]

Inflammation and the gut microbiome

Some association between inflammatory conditions such as autoimmune diseases and a decrease in the diversity of 'good' gut bacteria has been seen.[3] Furthermore, a decrease in beneficial gut bacteria can increase the likelihood of developing an autoimmune disease.[4]

A microbiome with a low diversity of bacterial species can disrupt immune function and increase inflammation. It is thought that inflammatory diseases may commence in the gut with an autoimmune reaction that progresses into systemic inflammation – so now let's take a look at the gut microbiome.

POINTS TO REMEMBER
- Inflammation plays a vital role in the development of chronic diseases.
- Poor diet (high in sugars, vegetable oils and processed foods) and lack of exercise are associated with chronic inflammation.
- Inflammation is associated with a lack of diversity in the gut microbiome.

The Gut Microbiome

A healthy gut means a healthy body.

Hippocrates is credited with saying 'All disease starts in the gut', and recent evidence suggests he may have been right.

Our gut microbiome (or microbiota), a term coined in 2001 by molecular biologist Joshua Lederberg, refers to the trillions of microbes (bacteria, yeasts and other fungi, and viruses) that live inside our bowels, interacting not only with the food we eat, but also with each other and with us.[1] Each person's microbiome is unique.

There are more bacterial cells in our own body than there are human cells (although not in a ratio of ten to one as was once thought, but probably close to one to one), and most of those bacteria live in our gut. There are more than a thousand different species of bacteria that take up residence in the human colon. These microbes aid in digestion, make vitamins and other nutrients, break down dietary toxins, strengthen the body's internal barrier against the contents of the gut, help prevent infection, and can also influence the immune system and our mood.

The digestive tract lining has a greater surface area than even our skin, and has three types of chemical detector – nerve cells, endocrine cells and immune cells. There are more of these detectors in the gut than in any other organ. The gut contains 70–80 per cent of all the immune cells in the body and nearly a billion neurons, and uses more than 20 identified hormones. The composition of the microbiome has a significant effect on these detectors. A healthy, balanced microbiome therefore has a profound influence on our overall health and wellbeing.

OUR MICROBIOME HAS CHANGED

A number of studies have shown that the bacterial diversity of the microbiome in Western populations has declined significantly in recent evolutionary history and has much less diversity than in traditional tribal populations.[2] This is a problem because people with lower microbiome diversity are more likely to show symptoms of inflammation and develop metabolic health issues such as type 2 diabetes. If they eat a better diet that increases their microbiome diversity, a lot of those markers get better.

There are a number of possible reasons for lack of diversity in the Western biome, including diet, hygiene and our widespread use of antibiotics. When we take antibiotics, our microbiome diversity is greatly reduced and then gradually rebuilds over the following weeks and months as the bacterial community recovers. Improved hygiene has had a dramatic positive effect on human health with a huge reduction in mortality due to infections, but our 'obsession' with hygiene may have reduced our exposure to bacteria and thus reduced the diversity of our gut microbiome.

Fortunately, improving the diet can increase microbiome diversity and lead to improvements in the conditions associated with lack of diversity in the gut microbiome.

The gut microbiome and fibre

The majority of the gut microbes are found in the large intestine or bowel (colon), which means they live on the parts of our food that are poorly digested – in other words, fibre from plant foods. Humans have no digestive enzymes that can digest fibre, so it passes through the small intestine unchanged. There are two main types of fibre:

- **Soluble or fermentable**: This is fibre fermented and digested by the 'good' gut bacteria in the colon (large intestine). As a result, a healthy population of gut microbiota is essential for optimal fibre digestion. Foods containing fermentable fibre include most fruits and vegetables, and certain whole grains such as oats.
- **Insoluble or non-fermentable**: This fibre is resistant even to bacterial fermentation in the colon and so passes out of the body unchanged. Non-fermentable fibre thickens stools and reduces the time it takes food to pass through the gut. This type of fibre is found predominantly in cellulose-rich foods, such as whole grains.

The suggested health benefits of fibre include improved blood sugar control, weight loss, better skin, and perhaps reduction in the risk of diseases such as heart disease, stroke, diverticular disease, irritable bowel syndrome, haemorrhoids, gallstones and possibly colon cancer.[3] Too much fibre can also be a problem, though: it can result in constipation, gas and bloating, abdominal cramps and dehydration.

The recommended daily fibre intake is 30 grams for men and 25 grams for women. Generally, a real-food, nutrient-dense diet will provide sufficient fibre in the best form, from excellent foods such as vegetables, fruits, nuts and seeds.

Is the microbiome the key to good health?

We've known for a long time that gut bacteria are important for gut health, affecting digestion and absorption, but the recent evidence seems to suggest that the microbiome also has a whole-body effect on the immune system and metabolism.[4] It also appears to have an effect on brain chemistry, affecting mood and behaviour.[5] Some have termed the microbiome the 'control centre for human biology'.[6]

There also appears to be a major connection between our gut microbiome and inflammation. Negative changes in the intestinal microbiome are strongly associated with metabolic and inflammatory chronic diseases, including inflammatory bowel disease, cancer, cardiovascular disease and metabolic syndrome.[7]

We now recognise that allergic disorders, asthma and possibly obesity are also related to an unhealthy population of intestinal bacteria. Even simple ageing gradually shifts our intestinal bacterial population towards a disease-promoting, rather than disease-preventing, state.

The gut microbiome undergoes many changes during our first two years of life. Research has shown that this pattern of development is altered in children who are delivered by caesarean section, fed formula or treated with antibiotics.[8] Caesarean sections can influence the microbial community that first colonises the infant gut. We don't know the ultimate effect on adult gut bacterial diversity, but this is something that could affect the succession and building of the microbiome as a baby is growing and developing. It has been suggested that taking a swab from the mother's vagina and applying it to the skin of the newly born baby, delivered by C-section, may improve the baby's microbiome. We also know that human breast-milk has important molecules, human milk oligosaccharides, that help fuel the microbiome, attracting bacterial species like *Bifidobacterium* and *Bacteroides*. Baby formula does not possess these compounds.

LEAKY GUT

The gut lining, the layer known as the endothelium, is just one cell thick. When intact and healthy, it absorbs nutrients from our food, and keeps toxins, undigested food and bacteria out of the blood.

We now know that certain factors, such as gluten and 'bad' gut bacteria, can lead to the release of a substance called zonulin, which causes gaps to open up between the endothelial cells and allows harmful molecules into the bloodstream.[9] This in turn triggers an inflammatory response, the common factor in all age-related diseases, and can lead to autoimmune reactions (the body attacking itself).

The gut microbiome and disease

Imbalances in the gut microbiome have been linked with mental and neuro-logical disorders, including anxiety, depression, obsessive-compulsive disorder and Parkinson's disease.[10] A study comparing the composition of the gut microbiome of people with a major depressive disorder and that of healthy controls showed significant differences. Decreased levels of one bacterium in particular, *Faecalibacterium*, were correlated with increased degrees of depression.[11]

Research also suggests that children with autism have lower gut microbial diversity, and lower levels of important strains of healthy bacteria.[12] These differences may play a role in behavioural symptoms such as impaired social functioning.

Studies with obese and non-obese mice showed a dramatic effect when the gut bacteria from a non-obese mouse was introduced into obese mice and vice versa.[13] This encouraged scientists to speculate that alter-ing the gut microbiome could be the secret to reducing obesity in humans. Unfortunately, the results of faecal transplants in humans have not been shown to be as dramatic, possibly due to our genetic diversity as a species.

How to improve your microbiome

There are two steps to improving your microbiome:

1. Remove the factors causing the damage:
   - remove sugar, processed foods and vegetable oils from your diet
   - limit the use of medications such as antibiotics and anti-inflammatories
   - give up smoking
   - reduce your stress levels
   - limit your alcohol intake.
2. Replace them with better alternatives:
   - plenty of real food, including vegetables and fruit, especially berries, along with nuts, olive oil, green tea and dark chocolate
   - probiotics (see below)
   - prebiotics such as asparagus, under-ripe bananas, eggplants, endive, garlic, onions, leeks, Jerusalem artichokes and legumes (beans, peas and lentils)
   - gelatin from animal bones and cartilage, found in bone broth and other foods
   - increased physical activity
   - sufficient sleep.

Probiotics

Probiotics are live microorganisms that, when consumed in sufficient amounts, provide a health benefit. Probiotics have formed a vital part of many traditional diets for thousands of years, including Mediterranean and Middle Eastern diets, in the form of fermented milk and vegetable products such as yoghurt and pickles. They are credited, in part, for the relatively low rates of chronic age-related diseases in those regions.

Beer and wine are fermented foods, as are sourdough bread, live yoghurt, sauerkraut, olives, cured meats, kefir (a fermented milk drink), lassi (Indian fermented yoghurt and milk), kombucha (a fizzy fermented tea), raw milk cheeses, kimchi (spicy Asian fermented cabbage), natto (Japanese fermented soybeans), Indonesian tempeh (similar to tofu), chocolate, coffee, miso, many cheeses and various kinds of pickles – 'all the really good stuff', as food writer Michael Pollan puts it.[14] These fermented foods usually contain strains of either *Lactobacillus* or *Bifidobacterium* bacteria, which make it through to the colon and improve the gut microbiome.

Ideally you would get your probiotics from fermented foods but, failing that, probiotic supplements are widely available. Choosing the best of the hundreds of different products is difficult. I suggest going for one with at least five different strains of bacteria, at least five billion colony-forming units (CFUs), no extra ingredients such as artificial sweeteners, and without an additional prebiotic.

Good-quality strains of probiotics have been associated with beneficial effects for some conditions, particularly antibiotic-associated diarrhoea, but researchers are examining a huge range of other conditions, from cancer to eczema – even mental health – which may benefit from probiotics. Proponents claim that probiotics can also improve high blood pressure, insulin sensitivity and non-alcoholic fatty liver disease.[15]

Most of the clinical research into probiotics has been carried out on unhealthy people. This means we don't know much about the impact that taking probiotics might have on generally healthy people.

Prebiotics

Not to be confused with probiotics, prebiotics are foods containing a type of fibre called oligosaccharides, which pass through the upper portion of the gut undigested, then feed and stimulate the growth of microbes further down in the colon. These fibres are also known as resistant starch. Types of prebiotic fibres that are known to alter the microbiome include:

- **inulin and fructo-oligosaccharides**: found in foods such as Jerusalem artichokes, asparagus, leeks, green bananas, chicory and onions
- **lactulose**: a man-made oligosaccharide commonly used to treat diarrhoea
- **galacto-oligosaccharides**: found naturally in breastmilk to help feed the microbiome of newborn babies.

Our gut microbes break down these prebiotic fibres into short-chain fatty acids. These, particularly butyric acid, are important for gut health.

POINTS TO REMEMBER

- The gut microbiome pays an important role in our health, and lack of gut bacterial diversity has adverse health effects.
- Diversity can be improved with diet, less antibiotic use, and eating both probiotics and prebiotics.
- The recommended daily fibre intake is 30 grams for men and 25 grams for women.

So now we've seen three different phenomena which all appear to have a major effect on our health: insulin resistance, inflammation and the gut microbiome. As we will soon find out, the same dietary changes seem to affect all three. Coincidence? It would appear not.

Now, before we get down to the nitty gritty of what we should be eating day-to-day, it is important to understand a little bit about the three macronutrients: protein, fats and carbohydrates.

Carbs, Fats and Protein: Getting the Balance Right

What they do, which we need and how much.

These are three major nutrients (called macronutrients) in our food – but only two of them are actually *necessary* for human survival:

- If you don't eat protein, you die.
- If you don't eat fats, you die.
- If you don't eat carbohydrates, you're fine.

Protein

Proteins are chains made of amino acids linked together by peptide bonds. When we digest proteins we break them down into their constituent amino acids. Amino acids can be divided into three groups:

1. essential: meaning we can't make them ourselves and need to obtain them from our diet
2. conditionally essential: meaning we can usually make these ourselves except in special cases, such as premature babies or the severely ill
3. dispensable: meaning we can synthesise them ourselves and don't need them in our diet.

The nine essential amino acids are phenylalanine, valine, threonine, tryptophan, methionine, leucine, isoleucine, lysine and histidine. The six conditionally essential amino acids are arginine, cysteine, glycine, glutamine, proline and tyrosine. And the five dispensable amino acids are alanine, aspartic acid, asparagine, glutamic acid and serine.

Protein foods come from both animals and plant sources:

- animal sources: red meats, pork, chicken, fish, eggs and dairy products
- plant sources: grains, legumes (beans, peas and lentils), nuts, seeds, and foods made from soybeans, such as tempeh and tofu.

How much protein should we eat?

Most authorities recommend that protein should make up 15–25 per cent of our total calories, with a daily intake of 0.8–1.2 grams per kilogram of body weight. This means a 75-kilogram man needs 60–90 grams of protein per day and a 60-kilogram woman 50–70 grams per day. However I suspect that many people would benefit from a higher protein intake, somewhere around 1.2–1.5 grams per kilogram of body weight. Certainly bodybuilders, strength-based athletes, pregnant women and teenagers going through a growth spurt need more. Interestingly, there is quite a lot of research evidence suggesting that older people need more protein.[1] One study showed that doubling the recommended protein intake to 1.6 grams per kilogram of body weight had beneficial effects on lean body mass and leg power in elderly men.[2]

It is important to remember when calculating your protein intake that a 300-gram steak does not mean 300 grams of protein; in fact, there are about 70 grams of protein in a 300-gram steak.

Can you have too much protein? That's a controversial topic. Excess protein can be converted into glucose via a process called gluconeogenesis, so some have expressed concern that this could lead to increased glucose levels in the blood.[3] This process seems only to occur when no other fuel is available, such as in people who are fasting or have no carbohydrate intake at all, so it is probably not a concern for most of us in our daily lives. However, those with kidney disease should certainly discuss their protein intake with their doctor.

Fats

Let's not confuse body fat with the fats in our food. They're not all bad, although some of them certainly are – just not the ones we've been told are bad for the past 30 years!

The different types of fats

There are different kinds of dietary fats, and it's important to understand the differences.

Dietary fats can be either saturated or unsaturated. In saturated fat, each carbon atom in the chain is bonded to as many hydrogen atoms as possible (in other words is saturated with hydrogen). This makes them less prone to oxidative damage and rancidity. Saturated fats are solid at room temperature.

An unsaturated fat has at least one double bond between two carbon atoms in its chain, and so cannot be 'saturated' with hydrogen. The unsaturated fats can be further divided into:

- monounsaturated fats: which have only one double bond in their chain. They're still relatively resistant to oxidation, and monounsaturated oils such as olive oil tend to be high in beneficial antioxidants and polyphenols, further protecting them from damage. Monounsaturated fats are liquid at room temperature. Oleic acid (from olive oil) is the most common monounsaturated fatty acid in the diet.

- polyunsaturated fats (PUFAs): which have more than one double bond in their chain. They're the least resistant to oxidation of all fats. Polyunsaturated fats are also liquid at room temperature. The most common dietary polyunsaturated fats are either omega-3 or omega-6 fats. The 'omega' naming convention indicates the placement of the double bond within the fatty acid molecule. Omega-3s have the first double bond placed three carbon atoms away from the omega end.

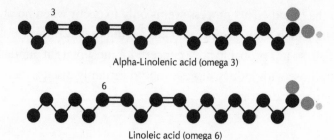

Alpha-Linolenic acid (omega 3)

Linoleic acid (omega 6)

Omega 3 fats have their first double bond 3 carbon atoms away from the omega end, while omega 6 have theirs 6 away.

OMEGA-3
Omega-3 fatty acids are a family of essential polyunsaturated fats that we must get from the diet. They are also called n-3 or ω-3 fatty acids. The three most important types are ALA (alpha-linolenic acid), DHA (docosahexaenoic acid) and EPA (eicosapentaenoic acid). ALA is mainly found in plants, while DHA and EPA are mainly found in animal foods and algae.

OMEGA-6

Like omega-3 fatty acids, omega-6 fatty acids are polyunsaturated fatty acids. The only difference is that the last double bond is six carbons from the omega end of the fatty acid molecule. Omega-6 fatty acids are also essential, so you need to obtain them from your diet. These fats are primarily used for energy. The most common omega-6 fat is linoleic acid, which can be converted into longer omega-6 fats such as arachidonic acid (ARA).

Fats and our health

For the past 50 years, saturated fats have been labelled public enemy number one, while polyunsaturated fats have been encouraged.

Dietary fats are a key provider of essential fats and fat-soluble vitamins, and all fat-containing foods have a mixture of saturated, monounsaturated and polyunsaturated fats – only the proportions vary. It is actually impossible to eat saturated or polyunsaturated fat alone. Dairy products are the only foods with more saturated than unsaturated fat. Many of the foods demonised by past research groups as high in saturated fats, even lard, contain more unsaturated than saturated fat. Sirloin steak for example is approximately 71 per cent water, 21 per cent protein, 3 per cent unsaturated fat and 2 per cent saturated fat.

Saturated fat

Saturated fat is found in animal products such as beef, lamb, pork, poultry with skin, butter, cream, cheese and other dairy products made from full-fat milk; and plant foods such as coconut, coconut oil, palm oil and palm kernel oil (often called tropical oils), and cocoa butter.

It should also be noted that processed foods, although they are primarily carbohydrate, all contain some saturated fats. There has been some confusion caused by studies of people consuming saturated fats within highly processed foods such as pizza, desserts, cakes, pastries, confectionery, potato chips, biscuits, pasta, bread, tortillas, burritos, tacos and hot dogs, many of which are high in refined carbohydrates. This has led to the false notion that 'saturated fat is bad', whereas the reality is that the combination of highly processed foods with any fats is 'bad'.

Contrary to what has been believed for decades, there is no convincing evidence to support the belief that foods naturally high in saturated fats are linked with heart disease.[4] In fact, saturated fat has numerous health benefits: it is rich in fat-soluble vitamins, and has been shown to raise HDL levels, reduce appetite, and promote brain health and even weight loss.[5]

Fats that have a high saturated fat content such as butter, lard and coconut oil are the best ingredients for high-heat cooking – much healthier than the polyunsaturated vegetable oils.

Monounsaturated fats

The body makes monounsaturated fatty acids from saturated fatty acids and uses them in a number of ways. Like saturated fats, they are relatively stable and can be used in cooking. They occur in olive, almond, pecan, cashew, peanut and avocado oils.

Polyunsaturated fatty acids (PUFAs)

Thanks to the dietary guidelines which have recommended replacing the saturated fats in our diet with PUFAs, as much as 30 per cent of the total calories in modern diets can be PUFAs, which is far too high. Our intake of PUFAs should only be about 4 per cent of calories, half as omega-3 and half as omega-6. The key to the intake of PUFAs is the ratio of omega-6 to omega-3 fatty acids. The ideal ratio of omega-6 to omega-3 is close to one to one and certainly less than four to one. Fifty years ago, the ratio in most Western countries was around one to one, but now the average is somewhere around 16 to one.[6] Unlike omega-3 fatty acids, which are anti-inflammatory, omega-6 fatty acids are inflammatory at levels higher than the one to one ratio with omega-3. And as we have seen earlier, inflammation is a key factor in a whole range of chronic diseases.

The omega-6 to -3 ratio has been further thrown out of balance by modern agricultural and industrial practices, which have reduced the amount of omega-3 fatty acids in vegetables, eggs, fish and meat. As an example, while free-range organic eggs from hens can contain one-to-one omega-6 and omega-3 fatty acids, in commercial supermarket eggs there can be 19 times as much omega-6 as omega-3.

Scientists at Stanford University analysed data from 19 different studies involving more than 45 000 people from 16 countries and found that those with higher levels of omega-3 in their blood were about 10 per cent less likely to die from a heart attack than those with lower concentrations.[7] Consumption of omega-3 fats has been shown to lead to improvements in the gut microbiome, which in turn is associated with benefits in obesity and type 2 diabetes.[8]

So we need to increase our consumption of foods containing omega-3 fatty acids while at the same time decreasing our consumption of omega-6 containing foods. The best natural source of omega-3 fats is oily fish, such as salmon, mackerel, herring, sardines, tuna and anchovies. I would recommend eating oily fish at least twice a week, more often if possible. If you can't manage that, you should consider a fish oil supplement (see page 159). Walnuts, chia seeds and flaxseeds are also good sources of omega-3 fatty acids.

Vegetable oils are the main source of omega-6 fatty acids, which are associated with numerous health problems. PUFAs tend to become oxidised or rancid during cooking, storage and processing.

TRANS FATS

A chemical hydrogenation process involving adding hydrogen atoms to polyunsaturated or monounsaturated oils creates trans fatty acids. While there are small amounts of trans fats in animal fat, most trans fats are found in highly processed foods. The chemical hydrogenation process in which hydrogen atoms are added to polyunsaturated or monounsaturated oils makes them solid at room temperature and less prone to rancidity, mimicking saturated fats such as butter and lard. During manufacture, some of the double bonds can change arrangement to form trans fats.

Partially hydrogenated oils are the major source of artificial trans fats. Recent science shows strong links between trans fat and a multitude of chronic diseases.[9]

In the US where trans fats are used widely in processed foods such as cookies, cakes, pies, and frozen pizza, their use is now banned. Fortunately, the amount of trans fats in the Australian and New Zealand food supplies tends to be quite low, comparatively. Nevertheless, it seems obvious that the government should be taking action to ban the use of artificial trans fats.

Fat content of common foods

It's all well and good talking about the different types of fat but we don't eat saturated, monounsaturated or polyunsaturated fats – we eat food. And food contains all three types of fats, which means you can't just avoid one type of fat.

Foods contain a mixture of all three types of fats

Food	Saturated (%)	Monounsaturated (%)	Polyunsaturated (%)
Almonds	9	65	21
Avocado	16	71	13
Beef	33	38	5
Biscuit, choc chip	35	42	18
Butter	68	28	4
Canola oil	7	64	28 (18 o-6, 10 o-3)
Cashews	20	59	17
Chicken breast	29	34	21
Chocolate bar	59	33	3
Coconut oil	92	6	2 (o-6)
Danish pastry	50	31	14
Egg yolk	36	44	16
Flaxseed oil	9	18	73 (16 o-6, 57 o-3)
Ham	35	49	16
Hamburger	36	44	6
Mackerel	28	44	28
Margarine	16	33	49
Milk	62	28	4
Olive oil	14	75	11 (10 o-6, 1 o-3)
Peanut oil	20	48	32 (o-6)
Pizza cheese	60	28	5
Safflower oil	9	11	80 (o-6)
Sesame oil	15	42	43 (o-6)

Note: o-3 = omega-3, o-6 = omega-6

Which fats should we eat?

For the past few decades we've been told to avoid saturated fats and replace them with polyunsaturated fats, but as we've seen, this is nonsensical. We should eat:

- foods high in saturated fats – meat, eggs, dairy
- foods high in monounsaturated fats – olive oil, nuts, avocado
- foods high in omega-3 PUFAs – oily fish, walnuts, chia seeds

and limit:

- foods high in omega-6 polyunsaturated fats – margarine, vegetable oils, processed foods.

The best 'healthy' fats	The best oils for high-temperature cooking
Almonds	Butter
Avocados	Coconut oil
Beef	Ghee
Cheese	Lard
Chia seeds	Olive oil
Dark chocolate	Tallow
Eggs	
Olives	
Salmon	
Sardines	

Carbohydrates

Carbohydrates are made from sugar molecules, and are separated into two major categories: sugars (simple carbohydrates) and starches (complex carbohydrates). Sugars contain one or two sugar molecules, while starches contain three or more sugar molecules linked together. In some cases, these chains can contain hundreds of sugars.

Sugars

Sugars can be monosaccharides (one sugar molecule) or disaccharides (two sugar molecules linked together).

Monosaccharides

Monosaccharides include glucose, which is common in nature. Also known as dextrose, grape sugar and corn sugar, glucose is the main form in which the body absorbs and uses carbohydrates.

Other examples of monosaccharides are fructose (fruit sugar) and the less common galactose, which is usually found as a component of larger sugars.

Disaccharides

Disaccharides, or double sugars, are composed of two monosaccharides. By far the best-known example of a disaccharide is sucrose, or table sugar, which is a glucose molecule bonded to a fructose molecule.

Lactose, or milk sugar, another disaccharide (this time of glucose and galactose), is the only type of sugar produced by animals rather than plants. Maltose, two glucose molecules bonded together, is the sugar in malt.

In Australia, sugar is produced from sugar cane, whereas in Europe and the United States, it's made largely from sugar beets. Sugar cane, a type of grass, is crushed to extract the juice, which is purified and boiled into a syrup from which raw sugar crystals are allowed to form. This leaves behind dark, sticky molasses.

High-sugar foods include:

- sugary drinks: soft drinks, cordials, energy drinks, flavoured coffee and tea, iced tea and cocktails
- desserts, cakes, biscuits, lollies and other sweet foods
- foods with added sugar, molasses, honey, and other sugars 'in disguise', especially if these are near the top of the ingredients list or more than one appears; 70–80 per cent of processed foods have added sugars. This includes many commercial sauces and marinades – yes, even the savoury ones!
- fruits that are naturally high in sugar, such as ripe bananas and figs, or dried fruit, which often has sugar added or is so concentrated by the drying process that it contains a lot of sugar.

Starches

Starches are polysaccharides (literally many sugars) composed of large numbers of glucose molecules bonded together, which means they break down into glucose during the digestion process. They are sometimes referred to as complex carbohydrates. Cellulose (a major component of plant fibre; see below) and glycogen are also glucose polysaccharides.

High-starch foods include:

- starchy vegetables: potatoes, sweet potatoes, corn, parsnip and taro
- flour and any food made with it, including bread, crackers, doughnuts, cakes, cookies, pastries (including gluten-free varieties)
- whole grains: rice, barley, oats, quinoa
- legumes: beans, peas and lentils (although these are more slowly digested, especially if the beans aren't tinned or puréed).

Fibre
Fibre, also classified as a complex carbohydrate, is the only type of carbohydrate the body can't physically digest. While this means it provides no nutrients to the body, it does perform a number of other important functions (see page 60).

TOTAL CARBS VERSUS NET CARBS
Some times food labels will contain the terms 'total carbs' and 'net' carbs. 'Net carbs' simply means the total amount of carbohydrates less the carbohydrate contained in the fibre. As fibre is not digested and therefore is not broken down to glucose with its subsequent insulin response, the 'net carbs' value is more relevant.

The glycemic index
The glycemic index (GI) is a measure of how 50 grams of a food affects our blood glucose levels after we eat it. The index works by setting pure glucose at the maximum 100, then other foods are ranked accordingly in comparison with it. A food with a GI of 50 raises blood sugar 50 per cent as much as pure glucose, and so on. The lower the GI, the slower and/or lower the rise it causes in blood sugar. By definition, a high-GI food has a GI of more than 70, a medium GI is between 55 and 70, and a low-GI food is less than 55.

The GI of a food depends on its protein, fibre and fat content, all of which slow down the absorption of glucose from the carbohydrates in the same food into the bloodstream.

The effect of high- and low-GI foods on blood glucose levels

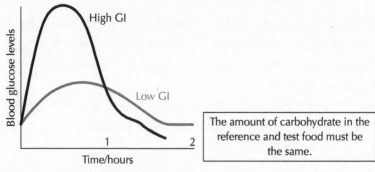

The amount of carbohydrate in the reference and test food must be the same.

Source: University of Sydney, 'About glycemic index', www.glycemicindex.com/about.php

Glycemic Index (GI) of common foods

Foods	GI	Foods	GI
Sugars		**Fruit**	
Glucose	100	Apple	28–44
Fructose	20	Banana	46–70
Honey	55	Grapes	46–69
Lactose	46	Oranges	31–51
Sucrose (table sugar)	60	Pears	33–42
Dairy		**Fruit juice**	
Milk (full-fat)	27	Orange juice	46–53
Milk (skim)	32	Pineapple juice	46
Yoghurt (unflavoured)	20	Tomato juice	38
Bread and crackers		**Vegetables**	
Baguette	95	Non-starchy	negligible
White bread	64–87	Carrots	30–47
Whole wheat bread	52–87	Corn	37–62
Muffins	55–80	Peas	39–54
Rice cakes	61–90	Potato	74–97
Crispbread	59–69	Sweet potato	44–78
Breakfast cereals		**Legumes**	
All-Bran	42–68	Baked beans	40
Corn Flakes	80–93	Chickpeas	10–38
Fruit Loops	69	Kidney beans	13–46
Special K	54–84	Lentils	18–37
Weet-Bix	61–74	Pinto beans	39
Quick Oats	66	Soybeans	15–20
Grains		**Nuts and snacks**	
Barley	22–48	Cashews	22
Couscous	61–69	Corn chips	72
Rice (white)	50–90	Ice cream	37–80
Rice (brown)	66–87	Popcorn	55–89
Pasta	40–60	Potato chips	42–57

Foods	GI	Foods	GI
Confectionery		**Soft drinks**	
Jelly beans	76–80	Coke	58
Mars bar	62–68	Gatorade	78
Skittles	70	Fanta	67
Snickers	55		

Why does the GI matter?
A high-GI food causes blood insulin levels to rise sharply, leading eventually to insulin resistance, obesity and chronic diseases. If you're going to eat carbohydrate foods, lower-GI carbs are much better for you.

Glycemic load

While the GI indicates the rise in blood sugar after eating 50 grams of a particular carbohydrate food, we generally don't eat all foods in similar quantities. The glycemic load (GL) factors in the amount you eat, using the formula:

$$GL = (\text{glycemic index} \times \text{grams of food eaten}) \div 100$$

A 45-gram packet of Skittles, for example, would have a GL of $70 \times 45 \div 100 = 31.5$. A baked potato would be approximately $85 \times 150 \div 100 = 127$.

Foods with a GL of less than 10 are defined as low-GL, medium-GL foods lie between 11 and 19, and high-GL foods are more than 20.

Which carbs are healthy?

Since the advent of the low-fat guidelines in the 1980s, carbohydrates have become our major fuel supply. We have been encouraged to eat bread, cereals, pasta, rice, starchy vegetables, fruit juice and other high-carb foods as the foundations of our diet, and many people are now eating 200–300 grams of carbohydrate every day.

I'm certainly not advocating zero-carb eating, but some carbs are healthier than others. Many foods containing carbs are full of other nutrients, such as vitamins, minerals and fibre. The table below shows healthy, nutrient-dense carb-containing foods divided into low-, medium- and high-carb content. Depending on your state of health and, in particular, your level of insulin resistance, you may need to restrict yourself to the low-carb list, or include some of the higher-carb foods once you have your insulin resistance under control.

Healthy low-, medium- and high-carb, nutrient-dense carbohydrate foods

Low-carb	Medium-carb	High-carb
Non-starchy vegetables – broccoli, spinach, cauliflower Low-sugar fruit, especially berries	Dairy (full-fat) Fruit – apples, pears, oranges Sweet potato	Cocoa, cacao, dark chocolate Legumes (kidney beans, lentils)

Starchy foods, such as potatoes, rice, pasta and so on are broken down into simple sugars by the body's digestive system before being absorbed into the bloodstream. Are they any better than simple sugars? Yes, because it takes time to break them down, which means there's no immediate surge in blood sugar and insulin response. They're still sugars, though, and have the same detrimental effect on our health, so they shouldn't be eaten in excessive amounts.

How much carbohydrate should we eat?

As I have said throughout this book, no single eating plan suits everyone, and yours should be tailored to your needs. Having said that, I think nearly all of us are eating too many carbs, and that cutting back is a good idea.

Carbohydrate content and insulin resistance with various diets

Diet type	Carbohydrate intake		Degree of insulin resistance appropriate for that diet
	Grams per day	Percentage of calories	
Standard Western diet	200–300	40–60	—
Moderate carb	100–150	20–30	Zero to low (insulin sensitive)
Low-carb	30–100	6–20	Moderate
Very low-carb (ketogenic)	<30	<6	Severe

Note: Figures are based on a daily intake of 2000 calories

As we saw earlier, your carb intake depends on your level of insulin resistance – or in other words, how sensitive your body is to carbs (see page 49).

Proportions of carbs, protein and fat

Diets are frequently described in terms of the ratios between carbohydrates, protein and fats – for instance, the 'Standard American diet' is 50 per cent carbohydrate, 15 per cent protein and 35 per cent fat, while the recommended low-fat diet consistent with the US *Dietary Guidelines* is 65 per cent carbohydrate, 15 per cent protein and 20 per cent fat.

A real-food, nutrient-dense diet would have much lower levels of carbohydrate (5–30 per cent), a similar amount of protein (15–20 per cent) and increased fat (60–80 per cent) of the healthy kind.

Proportion of carbs, protein and fats in different diets

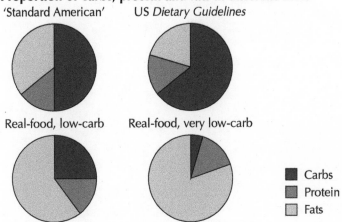

As we have seen earlier, the standard or low-fat diets have been a public health disaster associated with ever-increasing rates of obesity and chronic diseases such as type 2 diabetes. The emphasis on eating real food and avoiding processed foods leads to a diet low in carbs and high in healthy fats.

POINTS TO REMEMBER
- Proteins and fats are essential but carbohydrates are not.
- All foods with fats have all three types of fat: saturated, mono-unsaturated and polyunsaturated. Omega-6 polyunsaturated fats and trans fats are the most detrimental to our health.
- Most of us eat too many carbs. How much you should eat depends on your level of insulin resistance.

PART IV

My Five Golden Rules

Now that you have all the background information to start making decisions about what you should be eating, let me make it easy for you with these five golden rules. If you stick to them, you'll be well on the way to a healthier lifestyle.

1. *Cut back on sugar.*
2. *Avoid vegetable oils.*
3. *Eat real food.*
4. *Avoid processed foods.*
5. *Drink when you're thirsty.*

1. Cut Back on Sugar

Sugar is killing us and we need to do something about it.

The dietary changes we've made over the past 30 years have been a disaster for our health, leading to epidemics of obesity, type 2 diabetes and other chronic diseases. This has largely been due to our increased intake of two foods that are detrimental to our health – sugar and vegetable oils.

For many years, sugar was a luxury item – 'white gold' – enjoyed only by the rich. With the industrial revolution in the 19th century, sugar refineries could produce refined sugar in large quantities at a fraction of the previous price. This allowed the development in the 20th century of the confectionery and soft drink industries.

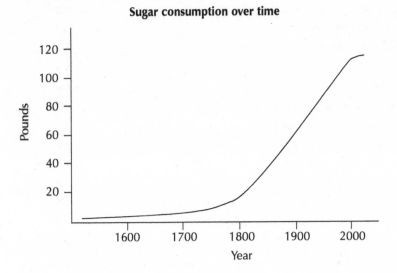

Sugar consumption over time

Source: Johnson, R.J., et al., *Am J Clin Nutr*, 2007[1]

How much sugar do we consume?

On average, each Australian has 64 grams (16 teaspoons) of added sugar per day. Teenagers consume significantly more.

In 2011–12, Australians consumed an average of 105 grams of total sugars per day. Just over half of this was free sugars (60 grams, equivalent to approximately 15 level teaspoons of white sugar) with the balance (45 grams) being the intrinsic sugars within intact fruit plus the naturally occurring sugar in milk.

Just over half (52 per cent) of all free sugars consumed were from beverages, led by soft drinks, sports and energy drinks (19 per cent), fruit juice and fruit drinks (13 per cent), with the sugar added to beverages such as tea and coffee contributing 7.3 per cent and cordials 4.9 per cent. At 14–18 years, the average daily intakes of free sugars were 92 grams for males and 70 grams for females (23 and 17 teaspoons respectively).

Consumption of added sugars among all Australians

Food	Percentage of added sugar intake
Soft drinks and flavoured water (not including cordials)	19.4
Sugar, honey and syrups	10.6
Cakes, muffins, scones, cake-type desserts	9.9
Fruit and vegetable juices	6.2
Chocolate and chocolate-based confectionery	5.6
Cordials	5.4
Sweet biscuits	4.6
Frozen milk products (ice cream, etc.)	4.5
Breakfast cereals, muesli and cereal bars	3.7
Other confectionery	3.0
Sauces, dips and condiments	2.7
Alcoholic beverages	2.6
Flavoured milks and milkshakes	2.5
Jam and lemon spreads, chocolate spreads, sauces	2.4
Yoghurt	2.1

Source: Australian Bureau of Statistics, Australian Health Survey: Consumption of added sugars, 2011–12, 2016[2]

Sugar-sweetened drinks

These are the major source of added sugar in the average Australian diet, especially among teenagers. In a 2011–12 Australian Bureau of Statistics survey, almost half (44 per cent) of all Australians aged two years and over had consumed sweetened beverages on the day before: 34 per cent had drunk sugar-sweetened beverages and 10 per cent artificially sweetened beverages (diet drinks).[3] In an average week, 62 per cent of Australian children drink fruit juice/drinks at least once, 58 per cent consume carbonated soft drinks, 32 per cent drink cordial and 29 per cent consume frozen drinks.

Within the Australian population, consumption of sweetened beverages increases with age from childhood, peaking in the teenage years, then declines among adults with age. More children (47 per cent) than adults (31 per cent) consume sugar-sweetened beverages.

The sugar content of common foods

Here are the sugar contents for the major processed foods and for fruit. You might be surprised just how high some of them are.

Soft drinks

The major source of added sugars, especially among children and teenagers, are soft drinks, sports drinks, energy drinks and flavoured water and teas.

Sugar content of popular soft drinks

Drink	Serving size (ml)	Sugar (grams per serve)	Sugar (teaspoons per serve)	Sugar (grams per 100 ml)	Sugar (teaspoons per 100 ml)
Coca-Cola	375	40	10	10.6	2½
Coca-Cola	600	64	16	10.6	2½
Sprite	600	61	15	10.1	2½
Fanta	375	42	10.5	11.2	2¾
Solo	600	72.6	18	12.1	3
V Energy Drink	500	53	13	10.6	2½
Red Bull	250	27	7	11	2¾
Mother	500	52	13	10.4	2½
Gatorade Fierce Grape	600	36	9	6	1½
Powerade Mountain Blast	600	34	8.5	5.7	1½
Vitamin Water Essential	500	27	7	5.5	1½
Lipton Ice Tea Peach	500	26.5	7	5.3	1½

Source: Sugar Shame[4]

Fruit juices and flavoured milk

Fruit juices and flavoured milks have always been thought of as 'healthy drinks', but they are full of sugar as well.

Sugar content of fruit juices and flavoured milk

Drink	Serving size (ml)	Sugar (grams per serve)	Sugar (teaspoons per serve)	Sugar (grams per 100 ml)	Sugar (teaspoons per 100 ml)
Orange juice	250	20	5	8	2
Apple juice	240	26	6.5	11	2¾
Fruit drinks	200	18	4.5	9	2¼
Flavoured milk	300	28	7	9	2¼

Commercial sauces

I found a 920 ml bottle of barbecue sauce in the fridge at home recently after the kids had hosted a barbecue. Out of curiosity I calculated the sugar content, which came out as 492 grams – or 125 teaspoons in the one bottle! I was so sure I'd miscalculated I double-checked. It may seem hard to believe, but most commercial sauces are high in sugar.

Sugar content of commercial sauces

Sauce	Serving size (ml)	Grams of sugar (per serve)	Teaspoons of sugar (per serve)	Grams of sugar (per 100 ml)	Teaspoons of sugar (per 100 ml)
Barbecue	25	12	3	48	12
Chilli	20	3	1	15	4
Satay	20	3.3	1	16	4
Sweet and sour	20	8.5	2	43	11
Tomato	20	5	1	25	6
Worcestershire	20	4	1	20	5

Fruit

The sugar in fruit is mainly in the form of fructose. The different fruits vary considerably in their sugar content.

Sugar content of fruits

Low-sugar fruits (1–8 grams per serve)	Medium-sugar fruits (9–15 grams per serve)	High-sugar fruits (>15 grams per serve)
Apricots	Apples	Banana
Blackberries	Cherries	Dates
Blueberries	Figs	Grapes
Grapefruit	Honeydew melon	Mango
Kiwifruit	Nectarine	Pineapple
Lemons	Oranges	Prunes
Limes	Peaches	Raisins
Raspberries	Pear	
Rhubarb	Rockmelon	
Strawberries	Watermelon	

How do I know how much sugar is in my food?

Australia's Nutrition Information Panels, which appear on the packet of all processed foods, have a list of ingredients as well as the amounts of nutrients (protein, fats, carbohydrates and sodium) per serving size and per 100 grams or 100 ml. The label states the total amount of carbohydrates and the total sugars, but doesn't differentiate between natural and added sugars.

The US recently introduced 'added sugars' on food labels, and I believe Australia should follow suit. You can find the added sugars in the ingredients list, but often under a different name (see Other Names for Sugar, page 312), and it's difficult to work out the quantities of natural and added sugars. It's easier with dairy foods: in a yoghurt, for example, natural sugars (lactose) will usually amount to 4–5 grams per 100 ml, so anything over this is added sugar.

For more on food labels, see page 151.

Natural vs added sugars

Fruit, vegetables and dairy products contain natural (or intrinsic) sugars and have the added benefits of vitamins, other nutrients and dietary fibre.

Added sugars, on the other hand, are devoid of the nutritional benefits of natural sugars and add unnecessary calories to a diet. Added sugars are the major source of sugar in the Australian diet and appear in 70–80 per cent of processed foods.

The various types of sugar – white sugar, caster sugar, icing sugar, brown sugar – are all similar in structure. White granulated sugar is one of the world's purest foods – it's 99.9 per cent sucrose, with all the 'impurities' such as minerals and polyphenols completely removed. Brown sugar is 95 per cent sucrose and 5 per cent molasses, which adds a toffee flavour and moistness but no great nutritional benefits.

Sugar by another name

Sugar is found in most processed foods but you wouldn't always know it if you read the food label. That's because food manufacturers disguise sugar in many forms. As you can see from the table of names on page 312, there are dozens of different names for sugar such as agave syrup, corn syrup and cane juice. A 2017 study of 215 popular ultra-processed foods in Australia found that 95 per cent contained added sugars described in 34 different ways.[5]

In the US in particular the most popular form of added sugar is high fructose corn syrup (HFCS) which is either 42 per cent fructose (HFCS-42) or 55 per cent fructose (HFCS-55). HFCS is much cheaper than regular sugar (which is 50 per cent fructose), and extends the shelf life of processed products. Recently the US food industry introduced a form of HFCS containing 90 per cent fructose, which is being marketing as fructose syrup to overcome the negative publicity associated with HFCS. I'm not sure 'fructose syrup' sounds much healthier . . .

Sugar and disease

We've established that it's not eating fat that makes us fat, but eating sugar and processed foods, which leads to a state of insulin resistance. The key to losing weight is reversing that state of insulin resistance, and we start this by cutting back on sugar. As we have seen, sugar is everywhere – we're in the midst of a sugardemic.

Sugar consumption is closely associated with levels of obesity and type 2 diabetes.[6] American studies have shown that consuming one US 12 ounce (350 ml) can of soft drink per day can lead to a 6.75 kilogram weight gain in one year.[7] The same amount of sugary drink per day increases the risk of type 2 diabetes by 22 per cent compared with drinking one can a month or less.[8]

As we have seen, sugar consumption can lead to insulin resistance, which is associated with the development of obesity and chronic diseases such as type 2 diabetes, fatty liver and cardiovascular disease. Studies have shown that people who obtain more than 10 per cent of their calories from sugar have a 30 per cent higher risk of dying from heart disease. Those who obtain more than 25 per cent of their calories from sugar have triple the risk.[9]

One sugar-sweetened beverage a day results in an average 20 per cent higher risk of heart disease.[10] Even moderate consumption of sugar for a short duration may cause substantial harm.

One study has suggested that dietary sugar intake may increase the risks of breast cancer, while another found that those participants consuming the most sugar (particularly sugar-sweetened beverages) had a higher risk of developing pancreatic cancer.[11] A wide range of studies also link sugar to numerous other chronic diseases, including Alzheimer's disease and fatty liver.[12]

Fructose brings its own problems. Unlike glucose, which is transported around the body to fuel the tissues that need it, fructose is metabolised in the liver. Excessive fructose overwhelms the liver's capacity to cope and localised insulin resistance develops in the liver. This leads to an accumulation of fat within the liver, the 'fatty liver' condition I described earlier.

Other effects of high blood sugar

High blood sugar leads to the formation of compounds called advanced glycation end-products (AGEs). These speed up the ageing process by causing tissue damage, especially to the skin.

Prolonged excess sugar intake leading to persistently high blood sugar is also implicated in chronic inflammation, which as we have seen can result in chronic diseases such as autoimmune diseases.

How much sugar is okay?

No one is suggesting zero intake of sugar. That's neither practical nor necessary. We should, however, consider sugar to be a treat rather than a staple.

The World Health Organization (WHO) recommends that we obtain no more than 10 per cent, and ideally 5 per cent, of our daily calories from added sugar. In a typical intake of 2000 calories, 5 per cent is 100 calories.

With each gram of sugar producing 4 calories, that means the ideal intake of added sugar is no more than 25 grams (6 teaspoons) – though the right amount for each individual is closely related to their insulin sensitivity.

SUGAR AND WEIGHT LOSS

There is plenty of scientific evidence to support weight loss by reducing sugar and starchy foods. I'm aware of 57 research trials comparing low-fat to low-carb diets for weight loss. Of those 57, 48 showed greater weight loss with low-carb than low-fat diets (most by quite large margins), two were equal, and seven showed slightly more weight loss with a low-fat diet.[13] The most recent meta-analysis comparing low-carb and low-fat diets concluded that, 'compared with subjects on low-fat diets, subjects on low-carbohydrate diets experienced significantly greater weight loss, greater triglycerides reduction and greater increase in HDL-cholesterol after 6 months to 2 years of intervention'.[14]

If you want to lose weight these are the steps to take:

1. No sugar-sweetened drinks – soft drinks, sports drinks, energy drinks, fruit juices – including sugar in coffee and tea.
2. No starchy foods – pasta, rice, potatoes – which are broken down to glucose.
3. No processed grains – white bread and bread products (muffins, crumpets, cakes, biscuits).
4. No foods with hidden sugars – flavoured yoghurts, muesli bars, sauces and dressings.

How sugar gets us hooked

Sugar activates the same dopamine reward system as nicotine and cocaine, which feels so good it makes us want to eat sugar again. This can lead to cravings and addiction.

When we eat a lot of sugary foods regularly, the body adapts to prevent overstimulation of the reward system. This means we need more sugar for the same hit each time. This may sounds similar to the development of tolerance in drug addicts, and it certainly leads to increased sugar consumption. Sugar addiction has not been scientifically proven, but it does have addictive-like qualities. Cutting out sugar is very difficult, and quitting 'cold turkey' leads to withdrawal symptoms that for some people pass quickly but for others are almost unbearable.

Using sugar substitutes is probably not helpful, as it continues our addiction to sweetness. (For more on sugar substitutes, see page 161.)

POINTS TO REMEMBER
- Most processed foods contain added sugars and these can have many different names.
- There are clear associations between excessive sugar consumption and obesity, type 2 diabetes and other chronic diseases.
- The WHO suggests that our ideal daily intake of added sugar should be no more than 6 teaspoons per day at most.

---

2. No Vegetable Oils

We weren't built to eat vegetable oils.

As we saw earlier, vegetable oils such as cottonseed, corn, soybean, safflower, peanut, flaxseed, rapeseed and canola oils are unsaturated oils, primarily polyunsaturated; that is they have multiple double bonds (the oils from linseed and rapeseed are blended to form canola oil) with some monounsaturated fats and a small amount of saturated fats.

The double bonds of these polyunsaturated oils can react with the air so the oils oxidise and go bad (rancid) easily. These oils were not as useful as solid fats such as butter or lard, so were not used widely until the process of hydrogenation was discovered, which converted oils into solid fats (see page 71).

The hydrogenation of oil was discovered by a scientist in Germany in the early 20th century and used by the US food giant Procter and Gamble to produce a hydrogenated oil they called *Crisco* – named after its content, crystallised cottonseed oil. Hydrogenated oils are used in the manufacture of thousands of processed foods. Highly hydrogenated oils are ideal for making chocolate coatings and hard cake icings, whereas a lightly hydrogenated oil is used in fluid products such as sauces or dressings, while an oil that's somewhere in between is used for creamy fillings and baked goods.

The other widespread use of these hydrogenated oils has been in the manufacture of margarine, which became widely used as a substitute for butter. A chemically created 'food', margarine was cheaper than butter and did not contain the falsely demonised saturated fats. Margarine was therefore promoted as the cheap, healthy alternative to the saturated fat-containing butter.

At the start of the 20th century, most of the fatty acids in our diet were either saturated or monounsaturated, primarily from butter, lard, tallow, coconut oil and small amounts of olive oil. Today most of the fats in our diet are polyunsaturated from vegetable oils derived mostly from safflower, canola, soy and corn.

Changes in fat usage over the past century

Added fats

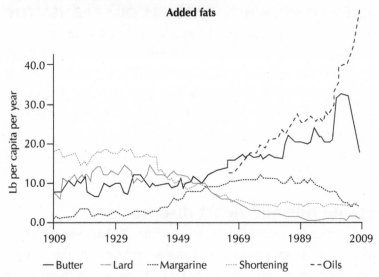

Source: Guyenet, S., 'The American Diet', 2012[1]

When saturated fat was declared the main cause of heart disease, nutrition experts advised us to avoid foods containing saturated fats, such as meat, dairy and coconuts. We were told to stop using butter and lard for our cooking, and to use the polyunsaturated vegetable oils instead. McDonald's, for example, switched from frying in beef fat to canola oil in 2004 and KFC followed suit in 2012. Vegetable oils are now the main fat used in almost all processed food.

According to investigative journalist Nina Teicholz, the increase in the amount of vegetable oils we eat is the single biggest increase in any kind of food ingredient over the course of the 20th century.[2] By one calculation, we now eat more than 100 000 times more vegetable oils than we did at the beginning of the 20th century. They now make up 5–10 per cent of all calories consumed.

The industrial processing of vegetable oil has been a major factor in the increase of chronic diseases in the late 20th and early 21st centuries.

> ## WHAT HAPPENS WHEN VEGETABLE OILS ARE HEATED?
> A study released in 2014 found that when polyunsaturated oils are heated to 180°C, a normal cooking temperature, they oxidise and form significant quantities of toxic aldehydes. If the oil is reused the concentration of these aldehydes increases. When the oil in the study was reused a fifth time, it had five times the concentration of these chemicals that it had on the first.[3]

Vegetable oils and heart disease

The huge increase in consumption of vegetable oils has led to an increase in heart disease. As we saw earlier, this was confirmed in the Minnesota Coronary Experiment and the Sydney Heart Study, which showed a clear link between high consumption of polyunsaturated vegetable oils and heart disease (see pages 22–23).[4]

How to decrease consumption of vegetable oils

Given all of the above, it would be prudent to avoid consuming of foods and oils high in omega-6 fatty acids.

The most obvious way is to avoid consuming vegetable oils. However, lots of foods are either made with vegetable oils or are naturally high in omega-6 fats. In a study of different foods and the balance between omega-6 and omega-3 fats, the food items with the most negative omega-3–6 score were:

Food	Negative Omega-3–6 score
Soybean oil	50
Mayonnaise	46
Tub margarine	39
Microwave popcorn	37
'Italian' salad dressing	35
Potato chips	29
Peanut butter	24
Tortilla chip snacks	24

That's basically a list of common junk food items. If you do nothing else but avoid those, you would be avoiding huge sources of excess omega-6 fats.

Overall the easiest way to keep vegetable oils out of your diet is to eat real, unprocessed food. Foods that are naturally rich in saturated fats, like grass-fed meats, grass-fed butter, pastured eggs and coconuts come in a near-perfect package, as they're typically loaded with the fat-soluble vitamins, A, D, E and K. Many of these foods also have a healthier omega-6 versus omega-3 balance.

Industrially processed vegetable oils, on the other hand, are highly processed and offer little nutritional value other than empty calories. More importantly, they can damage your cellular and mitochondrial membranes.

I no longer use any of the vegetable oils in cooking or dressings. Instead, I use olive oil in salad dressings, and cook with butter, lard or coconut oil.

POINTS TO REMEMBER
- Vegetable oils are widely used in cooking and processed foods.
- Vegetable oils are high in omega-6 fats, are oxidised into aldehydes and have been linked to heart disease.
- Use butter, lard, olive oil or coconut oil in cooking rather than vegetable oils.

3. Eat Real Food

Real food is the path to a long, active and healthy life.

If you start to follow the first two golden rules and cut back your intake of added sugars and vegetable oils, you'll already be taking some big steps towards improving your health and happiness.

We've already discussed the three different nutrients – carbs, fats and protein – so hopefully now you have a good understanding of the different ways in which they can affect the body. But we don't eat nutrients, we eat food, so it is time to start talking about food and what we should be putting in our mouths.

What do we want to get from what we eat? Food needs to be:

- . healthy
- tasty
- affordable.

It's important to understand the ratios of carbs, fats and proteins we need – which we've already covered – but a great way to think about it is simply: EAT REAL FOOD. Food such as:

- meat
- fish
- eggs
- dairy
- vegetables
- fruit
- nuts and seeds
- olive oil.

If we do that, and eat less processed food, we'll ensure we have:

- adequate protein intake
- fewer carbs

- good healthy fats
- no added sugar
- no toxic polyunsaturated fats
- no empty calories.

Let's look at these real foods one by one.

Meat

Meat has been an important part of our diet for thousands of years. It provides high-quality protein and some healthy fats, as well as iron and a number of vitamins and minerals.

Grass-fed versus grain-fed

Until relatively recently, all animals were kept in paddocks and fields on farms where they grazed on the grass. More recently, these animals are being fed with grains, either to top up on grass-feeding (called finishing), or completely grain-fed in feedlots.

The ratio of saturated to monounsaturated to polyunsaturated fat in beef stays about the same regardless of what the animal is fed. So whether your beef is grain-fed or grass-fed, you'll be getting about 40–50 per cent saturated fat, about 40–50 per cent monounsaturated fat, and somewhere near 10 per cent polyunsaturated fat. It has been shown, however, that grass-fed beef has significantly higher levels of omega-3 fats, antioxidants, minerals and other important nutrients – all good reasons to opt for grass-fed whenever you can.[1]

Quite apart from that, keeping cattle in pens is cruel. These cattle are also given antibiotics to reduce the inevitable infections associated with standing around all day in the midst of faeces and urine, and when we eat meat those antibiotics impact negatively on our gut microbiome.

The adverse health outcomes associated with meat eating are primarily around processed meat, which is probably not surprising when you see how the meat is processed – as my colleague Jason Fung puts it, 'If you knew how they made hot dogs, you wouldn't eat them.'[2] The other concern about red meat in particular is the possible connection with cancer of the colon. This is hotly debated, but it seems that, if there is a link, the problem is with overcooked 'charcoal' meat, so it is probably a good idea to avoid that.[3]

What about the red meat versus white meat argument? The recent trend has been towards increased consumption of white meat, especially chicken, but I believe there is a place for both red and white meat in your eating – both can be full of healthy nutrients. My major concern is how the meat is cooked – avoid using vegetable oils, so either grill or, if you're cooking the meat in a frying pan, use butter, lard or coconut oil instead. Think carefully about the sauce you serve with your cooked meat – most commercial sauces are high in sugar (see page 86) – and of course avoid the chips that accompany the meat. Just eat extra vegetables instead!

What about bacon?

Our grandparents loved bacon, but we have largely avoided it in recent years. It seems to be at the centre of the battleground between those who condemn it because of its high saturated fat content (although it's higher in monounsaturated fat anyway!), or because of its high nitrate content (not that high); and those who follow the low-carb healthy fat lifestyle, among whom it's one of the most popular foods.

So should bacon be avoided as it is a 'processed meat', or embraced due to its high fat content? Well, bacon is probably in a similar situation to other meats. It really depends on what the pigs were fed and how they were raised. Those raised on 'factory farms' and fed grains will be considerably less healthy than free-range pigs that grazed outdoors, got a lot of sunshine (which increases the vitamin D content of the pork fat), and ate a wide variety of natural foods. So try to buy bacon from pasture-raised animals. It's better to buy your bacon from a butcher (ideally an organic butcher) rather than the packaged variety at the supermarket.

Liver and other organ meats

Organ meats refer to the organs of animals that are consumed as food. The most common organ meats come from cows, pigs, lambs, goats, chickens and ducks, and include liver, tongue, heart, kidneys, brain, pancreas (sweetbread) and stomach (tripe).

In many ancient civilisations the organ meats were more highly valued than the muscle, which is the part of the meat that we like to eat these days. Organ meats have fallen out of favour, but there's no doubt that they're extremely beneficial for our health. My friend Zoë Harcombe, author of *The Obesity Epidemic*, describes liver as 'the most nutritious food on the planet', and she may well be right. It contains high-quality protein, some healthy fats, and is high in iron, folate, vitamin A and many of the B vitamins, including vitamin B12.[4]

Because it can take some time to develop a taste for organ meats, it may be best to start off with the more mildly flavoured organs, such as tongue and heart. You can also try grinding up liver and kidneys and combining them with beef or pork mince in dishes such as bolognese sauce. Alternatively, add them to a slow-cooked stew with other meats such as lamb shank. This can help you gradually develop a taste for these stronger flavours.

Many people find the taste and texture of liver unpleasant, but I often think it's more psychological. Liver can be eaten cooked on its own or added to casseroles and stews. Liver pâté is a popular way of eating liver from beef, chicken, duck and goose.

Bone broth

Our grandparents would use the remnants of the family Sunday roast to make bone broth and recently it has become popular again, especially among those trying to lead a healthier lifestyle. It's made by boiling bones to release nutrients, especially from the cartilage and bone marrow. Vinegar is usually added, and vegetables, herbs and spices can be added for additional flavour and nutrients. Commercial bone broths are available in both liquid form and powdered form, but by making your own broth you can ensure the bones come from good-quality beef (preferably grass-fed) or chicken. See page 303 for my bone broth recipe if you want to have a go at making your own (and don't mind the smell!).

There is little conclusive research proving bone broth's efficacy, but many swear by its benefits. Collagen, one of the basic building blocks of bones, skin, joints, muscles and tendons, is released into the broth from cartilage, as are other nutrients, such as chondroitin, glucosamine and hyaluronic acid, which have been shown to be beneficial in the management of arthritis. So it is important to use bones with joints, like chicken feet and beef knuckles. Chicken backs are also a great source of chondroitin and glucosamine. It has been suggested that bone broth also has beneficial effects for skin texture, the gut and cognition.

Fish

Fish, in particular oily fish such as salmon, sardines, mackerel and tuna, is among the healthiest of foods. You should aim for at least a couple of serves of oily fish per week – preferably more.

Salmon is one of my favourite foods. You can cook it in many ways – my personal favourite is baked in the oven with plenty of lemon juice, or you can add sesame and soy (see recipe, page 298). Salmon is one of the best sources of omega-3 fats, which as we have seen have numerous health benefits.

With Atlantic salmon we have a similar situation to beef: the salmon can be either wild or farmed. While both are healthy foods, in my view wild salmon is preferable, as it is free of contaminants commonly found in farmed salmon. Wild salmon has a darker red colour than the farmed version, which is more of a . . . salmon colour.

Sardines and anchovies are also a healthy fish option, as they too contain high levels of calcium, selenium and vitamin D.

Eggs

Eggs have had a bad rap for years and were probably the main victim of our cholesterol obsession. Now that it's been agreed that cholesterol in food has no effect of cholesterol levels in the body, we can go back to enjoying the wonderful benefits of eggs. It used to make me feel like crying to see people asking for egg white-only omelets when all the goodness was in the yolks!

Eggs are one of the most nutrient-dense foods, and arguably the single healthiest food there is. They contain protein, healthy fats, vitamins, minerals, various antioxidants, choline, selenium, vitamin D and riboflavin. I certainly try to eat two to three eggs a day, usually at breakfast, but I'm not that fussed about what time of day I eat them.

A study from Finland found that egg consumption was associated with a lower risk of type 2 diabetes as well as with lower blood glucose levels.[5] Men who ate about four eggs per week had a 37 per cent lower risk of type 2 diabetes than men who only ate one egg per week.

Similarly to beef and salmon, eggs from pasture-raised (properly free-range) chickens have an overall healthier nutrient profile, with more vitamins A, D and E, and higher omega-3 and lower omega-6 levels.

Remember, all the goodness is in the yolk, so please no more egg white omelets. And it's never too early to start kids on eggs – a recent study showed an increase in growth among 6–9-month-old babies that ate eggs.[6]

Eat your eggs with nutrient-dense, low-carb foods such as smoked salmon and non-starchy vegetables like spinach or avocado, rather than toast. The traditional eggs and bacon is a pretty good way to go as well.

Dairy

Although some argue that it's unnatural for humans to eat dairy beyond infancy – one of the reasons dairy is excluded by those following a Paleo diet – people in some areas of the world have been eating dairy for thousands of years and there are many studies that document how our genes have changed to accommodate dairy products in the diet.

For those who can tolerate dairy, it can be a very healthy food group. Studies have shown either a neutral or positive effect of dairy consumption in a whole range of health outcomes such as weight, heart disease and diabetes. A recent review of all the published research showed the higher the total dairy intake, the lower the incidence of cardiovascular disease.[7]

Numerous studies show that dairy products provide clear benefits for bone health at all ages, growing strong bones in children and helping us maintain bone density as we age. This appears to be due not just to the high calcium levels in dairy foods, but also their protein, phosphorus and vitamin K2 content.

It seems that consumption of dairy fat is protective to health, and full-fat dairy has higher protective health properties and benefits than low-fat dairy.

That's the good news. The reality is that many people do not tolerate dairy.

Dairy intolerances

There are two main groups who struggle with dairy: those who are lactose intolerant and those who can't digest A1 casein.

Lactose intolerance is a very common digestive problem, affecting about 75 per cent of the world's population. It's most prevalent in Asia and South America, but much less common in parts of the Western world such as North America, Europe and Australia. Those who are lactose intolerant don't make enough of the enzyme called lactase in their gut. Without sufficient lactase, lactose can pass through the gut undigested and cause unpleasant symptoms such as nausea, pain, gas, bloating and diarrhoea.

People with lactose intolerance tend to avoid dairy completely, but that may not be necessary, as not all dairy foods contain enough lactose to cause problems. Many people with an intolerance can eat up to 12 grams of lactose at a time without experiencing any symptoms. To put that in perspective, 12 grams is the amount found in 230 ml of milk.

Additionally, you might be surprised to learn that some dairy foods are naturally low in lactose. These include butter, hard cheese (such as cheddar, Parmesan, Swiss), probiotic yoghurt (best is a full-fat, probiotic yogurt that contains live bacterial cultures), kefir (a fermented milk drink) and pure cream or heavy full-fat cream (a high-fat product that contains almost no lactose).

The second group which is intolerant of dairy are those who cannot digest one of the milk proteins. There are two different forms of the beta-casein protein in milk – A1 and A2. A lot of people can digest the A2 form but not the A1 form, which they find inflammatory.

If you are experiencing inflammation symptoms such as regular involuntary sneezing, runny or itchy nose and eyes, skin blotches, rashes and/or eczema-like symptoms, then look closely at your dairy intake. If you suspect you're intolerant to A1, speak to your doctor and consider drastically reducing your milk intake, changing to A2-only milk, or dropping it from your diet – at least on a trial basis. There are plenty of milk and cream substitutes out there such as soy milk and coconut cream, which you can use in both tea and coffee.

Full-fat or low-fat dairy?

Now that we understand that consuming animal saturated fat is not a bad thing, drinking skim or skinny milk makes no sense at all. In fact, studies have shown you're more likely to gain weight drinking skim milk than full-fat.[8]

Yoghurt has traditionally been regarded as a 'healthy' food, but there's enormous variation in the content of yoghurts. The commonly eaten fruit yoghurts are high in sugar and should be avoided at all costs. You're much better off having a plain yoghurt and a piece of fruit than a fruit yoghurt.

The best yoghurt is a full-fat Greek yoghurt, which has a small amount of carbs (5 per cent) and plenty of healthy fats.

Butter is the current comeback food king. Having been replaced for many years by margarine – a foolish nutrition decision, we're now realising – more and more people are eating butter again and enjoying both the taste and health benefits. I use butter to cook with, and I put it on my meat (a dob of butter on a nice steak – beautiful) and vegetables.

As with beef, I always try to buy butter from the milk of grass-fed cows, which has more omega-3 fatty acids. Grass-fed dairy is also much higher in fat-soluble vitamins, especially vitamin K2, which is important for regulating calcium metabolism and so has major benefits for both bone and heart health.

Nutrient profile of dairy products

		Nutrient (per 100 g)							
Product	Calories	Water (g)	Carbs (g)	Fat (g)	Protein (g)	Vitamin A (IU)	Vitamin D (IU)	Calcium (mg)	Phosphorus (mg)
Cream	345	58	3	37	2	1470	52	65	62
Milk	60	88	5.5	3.5	3	102	40	113	91
Cheddar cheese	403	41	1	33	25	1002	12	721	512
Brie	334	50.5	0.5	28	21	592	—	184	188
Yoghurt	61	89	5	3	3	99	—	121	95
Butter	717	18	0	81	1	2499	56	24	24

Courtesy: Dr Zoë Harcombe

Vegetables

Vegetables are full of fibre as well as vitamins, minerals and phytonutrients, and are a vital part of any healthy diet. There's always plenty of debate about the recommended daily serves of vegetables – 5, 7 or 9? I think 5 serves – where a serve is 75 grams – is a good start, but more is better.

The only restriction on vegetables is for those insulin-resistant people who have to restrict their carb intake. They should certainly avoid the starchy group in the table overleaf and limit the intermediate group, depending on the severity of their insulin resistance.

Vegetables* classified on the basis of their carb content

Low-carb	Intermediate carb	High-carb (starchy)
Avocado	Beetroot	Parsnips
Asparagus	Carrots	Potatoes
Broccoli	Leeks	Sweet potatoes
Brussels sprouts	Onions	
Cabbage	Pumpkin	
Capsicum		
Cauliflower		
Cucumber		
Eggplant		
English spinach		
Green beans		
Kale		
Lettuce		
Mushrooms		
Peas		
Silverbeet		
Zucchini		
Tomatoes		

*Technically some of these are fruits

Fruit

Fruit has traditionally been regarded as a healthy food. We are told it is full of fibre, vitamins and minerals, and that we should eat at least two pieces of fruit a day.

On the other hand, fruit contains sugar. This sugar comes with fibre, a few vitamins, not much in the way of minerals, no essential fats and no complete protein.

The sugar in fruit is a combination of glucose and fructose. Ingesting glucose produces a surge of insulin release that then transports the glucose out of the blood and into the tissues. Excess glucose is converted to fat. Fructose, on the other hand, goes straight to the liver where it is converted to triglycerides, a lipid associated with the development of abdominal obesity, cardiovascular disease and fatty liver.

That explains why I am not as keen on fruit as many others: just because the sugar in fruit is 'naturally occurring' rather than added, that doesn't mean it's metabolised any differently. Admittedly, the presence of some fibre in fruit means that the sugar is absorbed more slowly, and it's harder to eat a lot, but it's still sugar! I certainly want to limit the high-sugar fruits such as grapes, mangoes, watermelon, pineapple and bananas.

The main fruits I eat are berries, including strawberries, raspberries, blueberries and blackberries, which are all relatively low in sugar. Even then I restrict them to small amounts. If you're insulin sensitive, one to two pieces of whole fruit per day, such as an apple or pear, is fine.

The things you *really* need to avoid are fruit juices (either commercial or homemade) and fruit drinks, where everything but the sugar has been stripped from the fruit, but it's still marketed as a healthy option. Dried fruit, where the sugar is very concentrated, should also be avoided.

There is, however, one fruit that's right up there on my list of favourite foods. Avocado is actually a fruit, but is unusual in that it's full of healthy monounsaturated fats with some omega-3 fats, making it a 'healthy fat'. Avocados can be eaten with any meal, either as they come or as a guacamole dip. Of course, 'smashed avocado on sourdough toast' has become the trendy thing to have for breakfast these days!

APPLE CIDER VINEGAR

Apple cider vinegar (ACV) has become very popular over recent years as a 'cure all'. However, it is nothing new – historical records indicate that apple juice has been fermented into vinegar for thousands of years, since before 5000 BC. For all that time, it's been used as a health tonic and remedy, including by Hippocrates, who prescribed it for coughs and colds, mixed with honey. Vinegar is also a natural disinfectant and was traditionally used in cleaning.

ACV may improve insulin sensitivity and glucose tolerance. Several small studies have investigated its benefits for people with insulin resistance, pre-diabetes and type 2 diabetes.[9] All vinegars (including ACV), when added to a starchy meal, reduce the load of the starch on the bloodstream, preventing the insulin spike such a meal usually produces.

It is important that you select organic, unfiltered and unpasteurised ACV to reap its many health and beauty benefits. Also, look for cloudy vinegar – this is the sign that the friendly enzymes and bacteria that promote healing have not been removed. The cloudy strands are what is referred to as the 'mother', and contain probiotics.

ACV has a bitter taste to some and should not be drunk straight. Dilute a tablespoon of ACV in a cup of water and if it is too bitter then add honey or stevia. Or simply use apple cider vinegar in salad dressings, or chilled vegie side dishes, like a vinegar-based coleslaw (see my recipe on page 301).

Nuts and seeds

Although some nuts are technically fruits, they're not sweet and are high in healthy fats. Nuts are high in fat (mainly monounsaturated), low in carbs and a great source of several nutrients, including vitamin E, magnesium and selenium, with many being high in fibre as well. Nuts contain antioxidants known as polyphenols, which may protect cells and LDL cholesterol from damage.

Although peanuts are technically legumes like peas and beans, they're often referred to as nuts because they have similar nutrition profiles and characteristics.

Nuts may help lose weight and lower total and LDL cholesterol and tri-glycerides while boosting levels of HDL cholesterol.[10] Several studies have shown eating nuts regularly can improve the blood sugar, blood pressure and other health markers of people with type 2 diabetes and metabolic syndrome.[11] Research also suggests that nuts could help reduce inflammation, especially in people with type 2 diabetes, kidney disease and other serious health conditions.[12]

Nuts can be eaten whole, as nut butters, or chopped up and sprinkled on food. They are sold in a wide variety of options, including salted or unsalted, seasoned or plain, raw or roasted. In general, it's healthiest to eat nuts raw or toast them in the oven at a temperature below 175°C. Dry-roasted nuts are the next-best option, but avoid nuts roasted in vegetable oils.

Almonds have the most fibre (12 per cent), and cashews and pine nuts the least (3–4 per cent). Chestnuts have the most sugar and Brazil nuts the least. Lastly, peanuts, almonds and pistachios have the most protein (21–26 per cent) and chestnuts the least (2 per cent). Brazil nuts and macadamia nuts (my favourite) have the most saturated fat, whereas chestnuts have the least.

Nutrient content of various nuts

	Nutrient (per 100 grams)					
	Calories	Fat (g)	Carbs (g)	Fibre (g)	Sugar (g)	Protein (g)
Almonds	575	49	22	12	4	21
Brazil nuts	656	66	12	8	2	14
Cashews	553	44	33	3	6	18
Chestnuts	213	2	46	8	11	2
Hazelnuts	628	61	17	10	4	15
Macadamias	718	76	14	9	5	8
Peanuts	567	49	16	8	4	26
Pecans	691	72	14	10	4	9
Pine nuts	673	68	13	4	4	14
Pistachios	557	44	28	10	8	21
Walnuts	654	65	14	7	3	15

Adapted from *Nutrition Advance*, http://nutritionadvance.com/types-of-nuts-complete-guide/[13]

Nuts are a very healthy snack but you can have too much of a good thing. It's probably best to limit yourself to a 30 gram serve (a small handful), which looks like this:

- 20 almonds
- 15 cashews
- 20 hazelnuts
- 15 macadamias
- 15 pecans
- 2 tablespoons of pine nuts
- 30 pistachio kernels
- 9 walnut kernels.

Seeds are also great sources of protein, minerals, zinc and other nutrients. I use them in my breakfast cereal (see recipe, page 293) and homemade carb-less bread (see recipe, page 295). My favourite seeds are sunflower, pumpkin, sesame, chia, hemp and flax. As with nuts, take care not to eat large amounts.

Olive oil

Extra virgin olive oil is mostly monounsaturated fat (75 per cent), with a smaller amount of saturated fat (14 per cent) and polyunsaturated fat (11 per cent). Extra virgin olive oil also contains large amounts of polyphenols, which have been associated with a reduced risk of several chronic diseases.[14]

This combination of healthy monounsaturated fat and polyphenols makes olive oil one of the healthiest foods around, and a staple of the Mediterranean Diet.

The word 'virgin' indicates that the oil has been extracted mechanically rather than chemically, and from the freshest olives. This makes it basically fresh olive juice, and the process retains the full flavour of the oil and all the healthy phenols. 'Extra virgin' should mean that the oil comes from good-quality olives, has no additives and has been stored to retain its integrity. Look also for 'cold-pressed', which ensures all the flavour and goodness is retained.

Like vegetable oils, some commercial olive oils are extracted using a high-heat chemical extraction process with solvents, and will usually be labelled 'pure olive oil' or 'light olive oil'. Some manufacturers have been caught out diluting their extra virgin olive oils with cheaper vegetable oils. It's safest to look for genuine seals of approval on the label, such as 'Australian Certified Extra Virgin'. If you want to test an olive oil, here's a handy trick: an unmixed olive oil will start to solidify after half an hour in the fridge, as it contains a large amount of monounsaturated fat. If it doesn't, it is fake.

MY REAL-FOOD LIFESTYLE

I try and eat grass-fed meat (including bacon), plenty of fish (I love salmon), lots of full-fat dairy (butter, cream, yoghurt, cheese), plenty of non-starchy vegetables, a bit of fruit (mainly berries), nuts (macadamias, almonds) as a snack, liver pâté, plenty of olive oil, and a cup of bone broth every day.

POINTS TO REMEMBER
- Food should be healthy, tasty and affordable.
- Eat real food such as grass-fed meat, fish, full-fat dairy, non-starchy vegetables, fruit, nuts and liver.
- Extra virgin olive oil is full of healthy monounsaturated fats and polyphenols.

4. Avoid Processed Foods

*Processed foods are packed with unhealthy ingredients
and don't nourish us.*

As you can see from the previous chapter, real foods are nutrient-dense and good for your health. The same cannot be said for processed foods, which usually contain empty calories, as well as significant amounts of our two main enemies – sugar and vegetable oils.

Processed foods usually contain one or more of the following:

- sugar (or sugar equivalents)
- unhealthy fats (especially vegetable oils)
- artificial flavourings
- emulsifiers.

'Processed' covers all foods that are pre-boxed or in wrappers, and includes processed grains:

- breakfast cereals
- baked goods
- chocolate and other confectionery ice cream
- cakes, biscuits and crackers
- popcorn and corn chips
- potato chips
- sugar-sweetened beverages
- diet drinks

- fruit juice
- margarine
- pasta
- pizza
- rice
- bread and grains
- honey
- commercial sauces and dressings.

> Beware of any food labelled 'fat-free' –
> that usually means 'high-sugar'.

Popular processed foods and healthy alternatives

Let's have a look at some of the more popular processed foods and come up with some healthy alternatives.

Pasta and pizza

These darlings of the low-fat high-carb dieters and carb-loading dinner of choice for the night before a marathon are full of carbs, which of course are broken down into sugar by the gut before being absorbed. Depending on your degree of insulin resistance you should either completely or partially eliminate pasta and pizza from your diet.

But you love pasta and pizza? Well luckily, there are tasty, healthy alternatives to both.

Healthy pasta alternative

Have you heard of zoodles? They're zucchini noodles (see my zoodle carbonara recipe on page 297). To make zoodles you cut the ends off the zucchini and feed it into a spiraliser. These can be hand-held or operated with a handle. (If you don't have a spiraliser, try using a vegetable peeler to create long strips of zucchini instead.) The zoodles then require a short cooking time in dry heat (i.e. you don't boil them in water like pasta). Cook them in a saucepan or frying pan for a couple of minutes only – leaving them too long or cooking them in water makes them soggy. Instead of zucchini you can also use carrots, button squash or any other vegetable.

Pizza alternative

If you love pizza, 'Fat Head' pizza may be your saviour. It was devised by the creator of the documentary *Fat Head Movie*, and the base is made using a mixture of almond flour, mozzarella cheese, cream cheese and egg. It's low in carbs and very tasty.

The internet is replete with other recipes for low-carb pizza base alternatives. Another option is a cauliflower pizza base, made using cauliflower, eggs and cheese. I've given you my cauliflower pizza recipe on page 299.

Rice

Rice is a very common accompaniment to many dishes, especially curries and Asian-style food. I'm happy to have a small amount of rice occasionally, but if you're insulin resistant and keen to keep those starchy carbs to a minimum, you should probably avoid it.

But fear not. Once again there's a healthy, tasty alternative: cauliflower rice. You'll find my recipe for cauliflower rice on page 298 – it's so easy to make.

If you are going to eat rice (and there is no reason not to eat small to moderate amounts if you're insulin sensitive), then which type of rice is healthier? Brown rice, black rice and wild rice are all healthier than white rice. White rice is more widely available on supermarket shelves than brown, black, or wild rice, and it's less expensive. However, brown rice is superior to white rice when it comes to fibre content, minerals, vitamins, and phytochemicals, and it often does not generate as large a spike in blood sugar levels after a meal.

Studies have found that eating white rice four or five times a week is linked to a heightened risk of type 2 diabetes, while two to four weekly servings of brown rice had the opposite effect.[1]

Breakfast cereals

Most children and many adults start their day with a breakfast cereal. These cereals are marketed heavily to children with free giveaways and dubious health claims. No parent concerned about the health of their child would give them dessert for breakfast. And yet that's exactly what most breakfast cereals are.

Here's a table of the most popular breakfast cereals in Australia from lowest to highest sugar content, with the number of grams of sugar per 100 grams, and the teaspoons in a typical serving (50 grams). Remember that the WHO recommends a daily sugar intake for children of no more than 6 teaspoons a day.

A child starting the day with a serve of Coco Pops or Frosties is already close to the ideal *daily* amount of added sugars.

Breakfast biscuits, which are basically breakfast cereal that can be eaten without adding milk, are becoming increasingly popular. Popular brands include Red Tractor, My Yummy Lunchbox and Belvita as well as the cereal equivalents (NutriGrain, Weet-Bix etc). These biscuits contain 15–30 grams of sugar per 100 grams, or 2–4 teaspoons of sugar per 50 gram serving.

Sugar content of popular breakfast cereals

Cereal	Sugar (g per 100 g)	Sugar (teaspoons per 100 g)	Sugar (teaspoons per serve (50 g)
Vita Brits	0.4	0.1	0.05
Weet-Bix	3.3	1	0.5
Corn Flakes	8.1	2	1
Rice Bubbles	8.7	2	1
Carman's Fruit & Nut Muesli	12.7	3	1.5
Special K	14.5	3.5	1.75
Cheerios	14.7	3.5	1.75
All-Bran	16.7	4	2
Sustain	19.4	5	2.5
Nutri-Grain	26.7	6.5	3.25
Milo Cereal	26.9	6.5	3.25
Sultana Bran	28.2	7	3.5
Just Right	28.7	7	3.5
Nesquik Cereal	29.9	7.5	3.75
Crunchy Nut	31.7	8	4
Coco Pops	36.5	9	4.5
Froot Loops	38.0	9.5	4.75
Frosties	41.3	10	5

Liquid breakfasts are also full of sugar. A 250 ml box of Up&Go, for example, contains 19.1 grams of sugar or 4.8 teaspoons. One box of Up&Go on the way to school or work and you're already close to your recommended sugar intake for the day! Up&Go also contains sunflower and canola oils as well as a thickener, maltodextrin, with an extremely high GI.

Just stick to real food. If you need some good breakfast alternatives, turn to the recipes on page 293.

Bread and grains

I don't know how many people, when I tell them I've given up eating bread along with other carbs, have said, 'I could give up everything else, but not bread.' Bread has long been known as the 'staff of life', and the Bible says, 'Give us this day our daily bread.' So why are we saying now that bread may be not so healthy for us?

Bread is made from a combination of flour, yeast, and sometimes sugar and salt. The flour usually comes from wheat, although other forms of flour exist – such as spelt (an older form of wheat), rye and barley. The problem is that bread is just not good for you. Dr William Davis, a cardiologist and the author of *Wheat Belly*, calls wheat 'the perfect chronic poison'. Or as Michael Pollan says in his book *Food Rules*, 'The whiter the bread, the sooner you're dead.'

There are two ways in which bread negatively affects our health. The first is that bread (and wheat and flour) is full of carbs and has a very high glycemic index, which means that eating bread causes a rapid spike in glucose and insulin levels with all the associated problems I have described earlier.

The second problem revolves around the hundreds of different proteins contained in wheat. The best known of these is gluten, which has glue-like properties (hence the name glu-ten) that are responsible for dough's stickiness.

I will tell you more about gluten later in the book, but a significant proportion of the population appears to be sensitive to gluten. Ingesting gluten gives them a range of symptoms including abdominal pain, bloating, discomfort and diarrhoea. Gluten and other wheat proteins may increase intestinal permeability (leaky gut, see page 62) resulting in an autoimmune response to substances not usually present in the gut wall and bloodstream.

The author of *Grain Brain*, American doctor David Perlmutter, suggests that the proteins in wheat have an adverse effect on brain function, which may be related to the gut–brain connection.[2] In his experience, removing gluten from the diet results in an improvement in symptoms.

Gluten is only one of many proteins contained in wheat and it is likely that many people are sensitive to various different proteins. By avoiding bread and other products derived from wheat products, many have experienced improvements in health.

There are plenty of low-carb breads available that are made from flour alternatives such as almond and coconut meal. Be wary of commercial gluten-free breads, as they often contain other high-GI starches.

The simplest gluten-free bread recipes contain almond flour, eggs and baking powder, although most are very dense. Adding the egg yolks and whites separately, then folding in the whites after beating, can help overcome that problem. If you want to bake your own low-carb bread, then I would suggest trying the recipe on page 295.

If you're insulin sensitive and can tolerate bread, sourdough bread may have some health advantages over conventional bread. Sourdough is an old form of bread leavening that relies on a mix of wild yeast and lactic acid bacteria, rather than added baker's yeast. Its lower gluten and phytate levels due to the fermentation process make it more nutritious and easier to digest. Sourdough bread also seems less likely to spike your blood sugar levels. Wholegrain sourdough is preferable.

Wraps aren't so great. Even though the fillings are often healthy, the wraps themselves are no different in their content from regular white bread.

But we've been eating bread forever . . .

If the human race has been eating bread for centuries without any ill effect, why are we having problems now? According to William Davis, wheat today is completely different from the wheat that was eaten years ago.[3] We used to consume ancient varieties of wheat such as emmer, einkorn and kamut, but most of the wheat eaten today is high-yield dwarf wheat developed by cross-breeding and genetic manipulation in the 20th century.

Dwarf wheat has shorter stems and a much greater yield, which makes the grain it produces cheaper than the older varieties and more economically viable. Wheat is also processed differently now. Since the late 19th century, milling techniques have made it possible to produce large quantities of refined wheat flour cheaply. In white flour, the nutritious components of the grain (the bran and germ) have been removed from the endosperm, where most of the starchy carbs are contained. This makes it much less nutrient dense and means it spikes blood sugar very quickly.

And we used to prepare our grains differently. They were soaked, sprouted and fermented, and bread was baked using slow-rise yeast. Sprouting and fermenting grains increases the quantity of the amino acid lysine, reduces anti-nutrients (such as phytate acid and lectins), disables enzyme inhibitors and makes the nutrients more accessible. Commercial bread is made with bleached flour and baked with quick-rise yeast. The grains certainly aren't soaked, sprouted or fermented.

As a result, Davis says, modern wheat is less nutritious than old wheat. The amount of minerals such as zinc, copper, iron and magnesium has decreased by a quarter. It also contains more gluten. Some studies show, for example, that people with coeliac disease can eat older wheat varieties without a reaction.[4] Relative to older wheat varieties, modern wheat has been said to have adverse effects on cholesterol, blood mineral content and inflammatory markers, potentially contributing to disease.[5]

All of this probably explains the widespread lack of tolerance to modern wheat. It takes generations for the human body to adapt to these sorts of changes.

Do we need to eat grains at all?

While there is no doubt that whole grains are better for us than refined grains, we might ask whether we actually need grains in our diet at all. The Dietary Guidelines have grains and cereals on the bottom rung of the food pyramid and want us to eat lots of them – but, as we know, those guidelines aren't to be trusted.

While whole grains certainly have some benefits, particularly as a source of fibre, they don't provide any nutrients that cannot be supplied by other foods. And while many people tolerate grains well, there is a significant proportion of the population who are better off without grains altogether. If you have some gastrointestinal (GI) symptoms such as bloating, or if you have been diagnosed with GI disorders such as IBS (irritable bowel syndrome) or GERD (gastro-esophageal reflux disease), then I'd recommend at least considering a trial of grain-free low-carb eating. I have had numerous patients who stopped eating grains (especially all wheat-containing foods) for a separate reason such as weight loss and then noticed their GI symptoms disappear once they got rid of the grains.

Flour alternatives

Flour is the basis of so many modern foods, it's hard to avoid it completely, but flour alternatives, such as almond flour and coconut flour, are good for cooking, and aren't associated with the same health issues as wheat flour.

Honey

I wasn't sure whether to put honey in the real food chapter or this one on processed food. An amber fluid made by honey bees from the nectar of flowers, honey has been 'nature's sweetener' for centuries and is frequently marketed as superior to sugar.

It probably should be considered as pure sugar, although the composition is slightly different. While sugar is 100 per cent sucrose, honey is about 75 per cent sugars, of which roughly half is glucose and half is fructose (depending on the source of the nectar) and the remainder is water with traces of protein, fat and fibre. This is why, weight for weight, honey has less sugar and calories than sugar.

One study found that eating honey for eight weeks significantly lowered LDL cholesterol and blood triglycerides, and increased HDL cholesterol, but increased levels of the blood sugar marker HbA1c, in people with type 2 diabetes.[6] Honey has slightly less harmful effects on blood sugar levels and metabolism than regular sugar.

There are lots of different types of honey. Monofloral honeys have a lower GI, and so can affect blood glucose and insulin levels slightly less. Creamed honey has been whipped to slow the natural crystallisation process, but has the same nutrition profile as ordinary honey.

What about raw honey versus normal honey? Most of the honey in supermarkets has been pasteurised (which means it's been heated briefly to 60°C and then cooled rapidly), then filtered, which makes it clearer and easier to package. This pasteurisation step stops the honey fermenting by also killing any yeast cells in the honey, and slows down the crystallisation rate. However, heating also reduces the honey's enzymes and possibly heat-sensitive antioxidants in the honey.

Many people believe that raw honey – with its flecks of bee pollen, honeycomb bits, propolis and bee wing fragments – is more wholesome and nutritious, but there is no hard evidence to suggest that raw honey is better for you than regular honey. If it is, the benefits are marginal and it's still sugar in another form.

For me, honey probably comes into the category of okay for insulin-sensitive people in moderate amounts, but definitely off the table for anyone with any degree of insulin resistance.

Sauces and dressings

Whether it is tomato sauce on your chips, barbecue sauce on your meat or mayonnaise on your salad, many of us use sauces, dressings and condiments extensively. The sauces are worse, though, than the food they accompany, and can turn a healthy meal into a very unhealthy one.

As we've seen, nearly all commercial sauces are full of sugar (see page 86). It's much better to make your own tomato sauce or mayonnaise – you'll find my tomato sauce recipe on page 304, and there are plenty of healthy recipes online. If you're looking for a healthier commercial tomato sauce, you might try one with no added sugar.

Chocolate

Chocolate, which I've included on the list of processed foods to be avoided, is a mix of cacao (or cocoa, which is cacao in its roasted, ground form), milk, sugar and butter. Cacao is rich in active ingredients such as flavonoids, theobromine and magnesium, which have positive health effects, such as lowering oxidised LDL cholesterol, preventing memory decline, and lowering the risk of developing heart disease and stroke.[7]

The trouble with cacao is that it has a bitter, unpleasant taste, so sugar is added to improve the flavour. Most 'milk chocolate' is high in sugar and low in cacao.

To get the positive health benefits of cacao, it's necessary to eat chocolate that's at least 70 per cent cacao and preferably even higher (85 per cent). Because of the lack of sweetness, there's no urge to continue eating, beyond the couple of small squares that are both tasty and good for your health.

POINTS TO REMEMBER
- Most processed foods contain sugar (or sugar equivalents) or starches, unhealthy fats (especially vegetable oils), artificial flavourings and emulsifiers.
- There are healthy alternatives to pasta, pizza and rice.
- Many of us are intolerant of modern wheat flour.
- Sauces and dressings are high in sugar.

---

5. Drink When You're Thirsty, Preferably Water

Water is the cheapest, healthiest and most satisfying drink we have.

We're all 60 per cent water, but we can lose water through breathing, sweating and expelling waste, and we need to replace that water, 20 per cent through food and 80 per cent through drinking.

If we don't replenish our fluids, we become dehydrated, with the potential for adverse health and performance effects. A common method for determining if you're dehydrated is to observe the colour of your urine – clear to very pale yellow urine indicates you're adequately hydrated, while yellow urine suggests dehydration.

There are two big questions regarding drinking: what to drink, and how often?

What to drink?

Let's start by listing what you shouldn't be drinking.

We've already discussed sugar-sweetened drinks such as soft drinks and sports drinks with their high sugar content. Unless you're performing high-level athletic activity, you probably don't need any added sugar in your drinks, so avoid the following:

- carbonated soft drinks – colas, lemonade
- 'isotonic' sports drinks – Gatorade, Powerade
- cordials
- vitamin water and other commercial flavoured waters
- fruit juices and fruit drinks
- energy drinks
- iced teas
- smoothies
- chocolate milk.

If you can tolerate small amounts of sugar, the following drinks may be suitable in small amounts:

- milk
- coconut water
- vegetable juice
- homemade flavoured mineral water (either with slices of fruit and fresh herbs added, or infused with food-grade essential oils to give off a fruity scent).

There's no question, however, that water is the healthiest drink, and most often tap water will do the trick. If you're concerned about the quality of your tap water, it may be an idea to install a filter or buy a filter jug.

If someone had said to your great-grandparents that people would pay for water in bottles and it would become a multimillion-dollar industry in Australia, they would have laughed in your face, and yet that has happened. In fact, with the sales of soft drinks finally starting to fall, the big drinks companies are looking to bottled water to maintain their profits and market share.

The most common complaint about water is its bland taste, particularly given we've been conditioned to expect sweetness in our drinks. A simple way of making water more flavoursome (and even healthier) is to add a couple of slices of lemon or lime, or some strawberries or mint.

Tea

Tea has been linked with a number of health benefits, including improved mood and cognition, and reduced risk of heart disease and type 2 diabetes. Researchers in Singapore recently found that regular consumption of tea brewed from tea leaves can reduce the risk of cognitive decline in elderly people.[1]

The health benefits and mouthfeel of tea largely come from three main bioactive compounds: catechins, caffeine and L-theanine. Catechins are polyphenols with antioxidant properties, caffeine makes us alert, and L-theanine, an amino acid, is believed to be what makes tea relaxing.

Whatever the type of tea – black, oolong, white or green – it comes from the same plant, *Camellia sinensis*. The differences come down to the time of harvest and the processing method, particularly the degree of exposure to oxygen. Black tea is fully oxidised, oolong is partially oxidised, and green and white teas are unoxidised. White teas come from early harvests, green teas from later.

Green tea has more antioxidants and less caffeine, which means it's generally considered to be the healthier option. Adding vitamin C, by adding a little lemon juice, say, has been shown to increase the amount of catechins available for absorption by a factor of more than five, allowing 80 per cent of the catechins to enter the bloodstream.[2]

When brewing tea, you must be patient. The longer you brew, the greater the concentration of the bioactive compounds, but the stronger the taste too. Brewing for 20–30 minutes at 80°C extracts most bioactives, but that's not a particularly practical approach, probably doesn't taste that great and will be rather cold!

Adding milk doesn't affect the health benefits, and there's no difference between loose-leaf tea and tea bags.

Coffee

Coffee is the world's most popular drink. According to estimates, we drink more than 400 billion cups of it each year. Coffee has high concentrations of beneficial antioxidants, phenolic nutrients and other healthy compounds. It's purported to have numerous positive health benefits including reducing the risks of developing type 2 diabetes, Parkinson's disease, Alzheimer's disease, colon cancer, asthma, migraines and liver disease.[3] Drinking coffee can also favourably affect markers for inflammation and oxidative stress.[4]

Caffeine speeds up the metabolism, which increases energy so you burn more calories.[5] In athletes, caffeine can improve short-term high-intensity exercise performance.[6] This same characteristic of coffee can, however, induce nervousness, anxiety and shakiness. People with an irregular heartbeat, high blood pressure or anxiety should probably avoid it. Too much coffee too late in the day can cause insomnia. It can also be addictive.

Don't undo the health benefits of coffee by adding sugar, and avoid coffee drinks like frappuccinos and flavoured lattes, which are loaded with sugar. Steer clear of artificial coffee whiteners (which will contain hydrogenated fats), and use full-fat cream or milk, or coconut cream for white coffee. Other healthy additions to coffee are turmeric and cinnamon. Bulletproof coffee, which consists of a mixture of coffee, coconut (or MCT) oil and butter, has become popular in the last couple of years, and may have beneficial effects.[7]

Coffee can interfere with the body's ability to utilise B vitamins such as folate, B6 and B12, which are important for mood regulation and during pregnancy. Pregnant women are usually advised to avoid coffee altogether or stick to only one cup a day. Overconsumption of caffeine has been linked with miscarriage, low birth weight and increased risk of cleft palate.[8] Caffeine also comes through in breastmilk, and an alert baby is not a sleepy baby!

A review of all the scientific research on the effects of coffee published in the *British Medical Journal* in 2017 found firstly that coffee was safe for all except pregnant women, and secondly that coffee consumption was associated with improved health, with the greatest improvement seen by those drinking three to four cups a day.[9]

Alcohol

Alcohol can have some health benefits when consumed in moderation (1–2 standard drinks per day), but many alcoholic drinks are high in carbs.

Dry white wine, red wine and champagne are quite low in carbs. Most spirits don't contain any carbs and are fine mixed with diet tonic or soda (but steer clear of high-carb mixers such as full-strength tonic water, colas and juices). Liqueurs like Baileys, however, are laden with sugar. Beer and cider are high in carbs, although some low(er)-carb beers are available.

Red wine has been linked with a variety of health benefits related to one of its ingredients, resveratrol. It's thought to reduce the risk of heart disease, raise HDL cholesterol and slow age-related mental decline.[10] In one study, people who drank two glasses of red wine a day had a better balance of gut bacteria.[11] The same study also showed that red wine drinkers had lower blood pressure, triglycerides, LDL cholesterol and the inflammation marker CRP.

Of course, drinking too much alcohol of any kind can have extremely negative health consequences.

Carb content of alcoholic drinks (standard serves)

Alcoholic beverage	Carbs per standard drink (g)
Champagne	1
Red wine	2–4
White wine (dry, e.g. chardonnay)	2–4
White wine (sweet, e.g. riesling)	6–8
Rosé wine	7
Port	8
Beer (full-strength)	9–14
Beer (low-carb)	1–4
Cider (sweet)	21
Cider (dry)	8
Whisky, brandy, gin, rum, tequila	0
Gin and tonic	16
Rum and Coke	39
Vodka, lime and soda	0
Vodka and orange juice	28
Margarita	8
Dry martini	0
Baileys	7
Jägermeister	11
Bacardi Breezer	39
Smirnoff Ice	38

How much fluid should I drink, and how often?

Australia's current dietary guidelines don't recommend a specific amount of water, but simply recommend we 'drink plenty of water'. The Nutrient Reference Values suggest a daily fluid intake from drinks of 2.6 litres (10 cups) for men and 2.1 litres (8 cups) for women.[12] Pregnant and lactating women should have an extra 200–500 mls a day.

We do have a natural thirst mechanism, although in recent times we've been told that by the time we realise we're thirsty it's too late and that we should drink before we're thirsty. This advice has led to episodes in athletes of exercise-associated hyponatremia (EAH), where drinking water dilutes their body fluids and reduces sodium to dangerous levels. After a number of deaths from EAH, a US consensus conference recommended that we should use our innate thirst mechanism.

Obviously, we need to increase our fluid consumption in certain situations, such as endurance exercise in hot conditions, but thirst will be a good indicator here too. The body is very good at adapting to our fluid status. When our fluids start to become depleted, the body secretes an anti-diuretic hormone, which decreases urine production and thus fluid losses. If the fluid depletion continues, we become thirsty.

> Let thirst be the guide to when you should drink, unless your GP advises you to increase your fluid intake for medical reasons.

MY DRINKING HABITS

I mainly drink tap water, coffee (flat whites), green tea, bone broth and the occasional glass or two of red wine. I drink when I'm thirsty, and on an average day probably drink 5–6 metric cups a day, which is 1.25–1.5 litres. On hot days and after exercise I drink more.

POINTS TO REMEMBER
- Water is the best drink. Let thirst determine how much you drink.
- Avoid sugar-sweetened beverages such as soft drinks, cordials and fruit juices.
- Tea and coffee are thought to have some health benefits.

PART V

How to Eat Well for Life

Enough of the theory – now it's time to look at what we should be eating. I'll take you through the broad principles before looking at some common dietary needs, from vegan and vegetarian to healthy eating for women and kids.

The Trouble with Weight-loss Diets

*A real-food lifestyle provides lasting benefits
a weight-loss diet can never provide.*

As I stated in the introduction, this is not a diet book. That is because 'diets' tend to be short term or temporary. We need long-term lifestyle habits, not short-term diets.

For many years pretty much everyone agreed that low-fat, reduced-calorie eating was the way to go. In recent years that mantra has been challenged, and now there are numerous diets claiming to be the one true way to weight loss and optimal health: Atkins, LCHF, Paleo, Mediterranean, Dukan, Sonoma, DASH, Mind, and so on.

So many diets, so much confusion.

Why do people go on diets?

The most common reason is for weight loss, but other motivating factors can be health issues such as high blood pressure, high cholesterol or cardiovascular disease. Many of these diets get a lot of publicity, usually promoted by a diet 'guru' or a celebrity.

There are literally hundreds of diets out there. Broadly we can divide them up into a number of categories, although some diets have elements of more than one, and therefore straddle the categories:

- low-calorie – Weight Watchers, Jenny Craig, SlimFast
- standard low-fat – Dr Oz, Zone
- low-fat whole foods – Mediterranean, Pritikin, Sonoma
- low-carb – Atkins, low-carb high-fat (LHCF)/Banting, ketogenic, Protein Power, Sugar Busters
- low-GI – South Beach
- paleo – Paleo diet, Primal Blueprint, Paleo Solution, raw food
- food-sensitivity – gluten-free, low-FODMAPs
- fasting – intermittent fasting, 5:2.

What do you want from a diet?

1. Achieve your goal e.g. weight loss
2. Easy to follow
3. Not too costly
4. Enjoyable food
5. Sustainable long term

Do diets work?

Most diets result in short-term (up to six months) weight loss, but 97 per cent of those who lose weight put that weight back on within 12 months.[1] Not only do they regain all the weight they have lost, as many as two thirds regain more weight than they lost over four to five years.[2] For many people desperate to lose weight, dieting follows a cyclical pattern over many years: restrict, regain, gain extra; restrict, regain, gain extra; and so on. The reasons for this are complex and multiple, but include increased hunger and a slowing of the metabolism in response to food deprivation.[3]

The body adjusts to reduced calorie intake by lowering its resting energy expenditure (REE), the energy that we use when at rest. When people find that they can no longer tolerate the deprivation/starvation involved in a calorie-deficit diet and return to eating as they did before, their total energy requirement (REE plus energy needed for activity) is lower and thus they regain weight.

Hunger is a huge issue for dieters, and is one of the main reasons the low-calorie and low-fat approaches don't work in the long term. From my own experience, the low-carb, healthy-fat diets result in significantly reduced hunger, which makes long-term sustainability much easier.

HUNGER AND SATIETY

Most diets fail because the dieter is always hungry. It's very difficult to stick to a low-calorie, low-fat diet because of the constant hunger. Satiety – the feeling of fullness after you've eaten – is a key factor in a healthy way of eating. It's not just the feeling straight after you've eaten, but how long that feeling lasts.

When we eat a meal full of sugars and processed foods, we may feel full at the end of the meal but this won't last long.

The brief surge in blood glucose leads to a spike of insulin production, which takes the glucose into the tissues, leaving the blood glucose level low again. And when our blood glucose drops, our brain tells us it's time to eat.

On the other hand, if we eat healthy nutrient-dense, lower carb foods, the rise in blood sugar is slow, without a big spike and subsequent drop. So the secrets of satiety (and thus maintaining a healthy lifestyle) are:

1. Eat nutrient-dense real foods (see page 96).
2. Avoid sugars and highly processed foods.
3. Eat slowly.
4. Focus on eating – no TV, computer, phone.

Portion control

Research has shown that portion size has increased in most Western countries, especially in takeaway and fast-food restaurants.[4] There's also convincing evidence that people eat more if portion sizes are larger.[5]

The contribution of increased portion size to the obesity epidemic is much debated, but if the increased proportions are high in the poor-quality, highly processed carbohydrates frequently found in fast food, then it's likely to be significant.

My freedom from hunger

As I mentioned at the start of this book, the first thing I noticed when I changed to eating nutrient-dense real food was a big reduction in appetite. I felt full for longer and went from constantly feeling hungry to virtually never being hungry. I went from three big meals and a couple of snacks (muffins, muesli bars), to two meals a day with occasional snacks (nuts or cheese).

POINTS TO REMEMBER
- Most diets have some initial success but ultimately fail.
- After a reduced-calorie diet, dieters regain their weight due to a decrease in resting energy expenditure.

Red, Amber and Green Foods

A quick-reference list for eating well.

I hope by now you have come to realise that what we eat has a massive impact on our health. And what we have been eating for the past 40 years has been all wrong! Removing animal sources of saturated fat (meat, dairy, eggs) and replacing them with sugar, vegetable oils and highly processed foods has been a disaster for our health – leading to obesity, type 2 diabetes, dental cavities, cardiovascular disease and numerous other chronic diseases.

In order to avoid or potentially even reverse these health issues, we need a real-food, nutrient-dense way of eating that is simple, affordable and enjoyable. To help you with this, I have divided foods up into three categories – those foods we can:

1. eat little of (red)
2. eat some of (amber)
3. eat plenty of (green)

The first and last categories are pretty simple; the middle one is the tricky one. As there is no one 'diet' for everyone, the amount of food you eat from the amber group should depend on the state of your health and in particular your degree of insulin resistance. If you're insulin sensitive (i.e. you metabolise carbohydrates well), you're a healthy weight and you have no chronic diseases, you can eat moderate amounts of the foods in the amber group.

If, however, you're at the other end of the insulin scale and quite insulin resistant, with excess weight, metabolic syndrome or pre-diabetes, high blood pressure, type 2 diabetes or any of the chronic diseases mentioned previously, you should restrict the foods in the amber group.

By now you should pretty much be able to guess which food is in which category. Sugars, vegetable oils and highly processed foods will be in the Red Zone; meat, dairy, fish, eggs, vegetables, nuts and olive oil in the Green Zone; and the rest in the Amber Zone.

Red Zone
Eat little of:

- Sugar – soft drinks, confectionery, chocolate, cakes, biscuits, pastries, ice cream
- Breakfast cereals
- Bread and related products (crumpets, muffins)
- Rice, rice cakes
- Pasta, pizza, noodles
- Margarine
- Flavoured or frozen yoghurts
- Fruits with high sugar/starch content – mango, pineapple, banana, grapes
- Dried fruits
- Muesli bars, low-fat energy bars
- Highly processed meats – hot dogs, nuggets, Spam
- Fruit juices, cordials, sports drinks, energy drinks, flavoured milks
- Alcohol – dessert wines, liqueurs, sugary mixers (tonic water, colas, lemonade)
- Artificial sweeteners
- Anything deep-fried in seed oils.

Don't cook with:

- Vegetable oils – canola, sunflower, safflower, cottonseed, rapeseed oil.

Amber Zone*
Eat some of:

- Starchy vegetables – pumpkin, potatoes, sweet potatoes, corn on the cob, butternut squash
- Most fruits – apples, apricots, peaches, pears, lemons, limes, oranges
- Nuts – cashews, chestnuts, pistachios
- Beans and legumes – kidney beans, lentils, peanuts, tofu
- Dairy – full-fat milk
- Soy milk, rice milk
- Low-carb energy bars

- Commercial sauces – tomato sauce/relish, barbecue sauces, chutney
- Alcohol – beer (preferably low-carb), red or white wine, spirits (avoid high-sugar mixers)
- Diet drinks.

*The amount you should eat from this group depends on your degree of insulin resistance.

Green Zone

Eat plenty of:

- Eggs
- Meat – beef, lamb, pork, chicken (preferably grass-fed, not grain-fed)
- Natural and cured meats – pancetta, prosciutto, bacon, salami
- Organ meats – liver, brains, kidneys, heart
- Fish – especially cold-water fish (salmon, sardines)
- Vegetables that grow above ground – including cabbage, cauliflower, broccoli, Brussels sprouts, asparagus, zucchini, eggplant, olives, spinach, silverbeet, mushrooms, cucumber, lettuce, onions, capsicums, tomatoes
- Avocados
- Berries – strawberries, raspberries, blackberries, blueberries
- Dairy products – cream, butter, cheese, cottage cheese, Greek yoghurt
- Non-dairy alternatives – coconut milk/cream, nut butters (e.g. almond, macadamia)
- Drinks – water, coffee, tea, bone broth, soda water
- Nuts – almonds, walnuts, Brazil nuts, hazelnuts, macadamias, pecans
- Seeds – flax, chia, pumpkin, sunflower and sesame seeds
- Olive oil and vinegar salad dressings
- Sauces – egg-yolk mayonnaise, mustard, pesto
- Flour alternatives – nut flours (almond, coconut)
- Fermented foods – kimchi, kombucha, true pickles, sauerkraut
- All spices, herbs, lemon and lime juice
- Natural sweeteners – stevia, xylitol, erythritol (see page 165)
- Dark chocolate – 70+ per cent cocoa.

Cook with:

- Butter, lard, tallow, ghee (preferably grass-fed)
- Olive oil
- Coconut, avocado and nut-based oils.

A new food pyramid

Earlier in the book I described the original food pyramid produced by the USDA in 1992. This became very popular and was constantly referred to as the definitive way to eat.

That pyramid was of course based on the obsession at the time with a low-fat, high-carb diet and encouraged the intake of grains while discouraging meat and dairy products.

The authorities have fiddled around with the food pyramid over time, but I quite like this one:

Healthy Food Pyramid

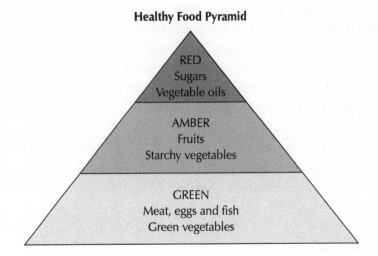

Breakfast, Lunch and Dinner Ideas

Try these suggestions for satisfying, long-acting meals.

Eating three meals a day is a custom that originated in Europe in the Middle Ages and has been exported throughout the world, in many cases replacing indigenous customs, many of which involved eating when driven by hunger or food availability, and so less regularly.

But is it necessary to eat three meals a day and, more importantly, is it the best regime for our health? As we've seen, in addition to those three meals a day, more and more people are now snacking between meals, usually on a highly processed snack full of sugar.

Since I adopted my low-carb lifestyle with more healthy fats, my appetite has dropped dramatically and I now generally eat two meals a day. The timing of those meals varies depending on my hunger and other social commitments. If I'm meeting someone for lunch, I skip breakfast, for example.

Let's assume we're eating three meals a day. What should we be eating? Here are my suggestions for breakfast, lunch, dinner and snacks. My favourite recipes for these meals can be found at the end of the book (page 293).

Breakfast

Breakfast has always been considered 'the most important meal of the day', but there's no scientific evidence to back up that statement. I suspect that is a marketing ploy by the breakfast food industry! In fact, breakfast is not essential and you can certainly skip it. And if you do have it, it doesn't have to be first thing in the morning – if you're not hungry early in the morning, you can eat 'breakfast' any time.

The content of the average Australian breakfast has changed dramatically in my lifetime. Whereas back in the 1950s and 1960s most people had cooked breakfasts in the form of porridge and/or eggs and bacon, in recent years, due to convenience, time constraints and clever marketing, we've been convinced to have a breakfast typically consisting of cereal with low-fat milk, fruit juice, toast with margarine and a spread, and tea or coffee. Low-fat fruit yoghurts are also popular.

And what's the main ingredient of that breakfast? Sugar.

I have two different types of breakfast, my quick and my big. Which one I choose depends on various factors such as time, availability or often just what I feel like on a given day. Both are filled with healthy fats and protein, which has the effect of making me feel very full. After one of those breakfasts I'm not hungry for a number of hours, which means I usually skip lunch and have my next meal at dinnertime.

My quick breakfast

For my quick breakfast I make up a mixture of nuts and seeds and add full-fat Greek yoghurt, some berries (depending on availability) and a sprinkling of cinnamon on top. I avoid the processed grains and high sugar content of breakfast cereals and mueslis (see page 112), and also avoid whole grains such as oats and wheat.

Nuts	Seeds
Almonds	Chia seeds
Hazelnuts	Coconut flakes
Macadamias	Flaxseed
Pistachios	Pumpkin seeds
Walnuts	Psyllium husks
	Sunflower seeds

You can either have the nuts and seeds raw, or combine them and bake them as in my muesli recipe (page 293).

My big breakfast

Eggs are the basis of my big breakfast. My favourite is scrambled, but I'm happy to go with poached, fried, boiled or an omelet. I usually scramble two or three eggs and eat them with some mixture of bacon or smoked salmon, mushrooms, tomatoes and/or avocado. If I had to pick a fave then I would say three scrambled eggs with smoked salmon and avocado. And no toast!

Lunch

If I'm having lunch and I haven't had breakfast, I'll often choose an egg-based meal such as an omelet with lots of vegetables, such as mushrooms, capsicum and so on.

Healthy lunch choices can be quite difficult, especially if you're trying to limit carbs, as bread and similar products are the basis of most lunches. Here are some of my other go-to options:

- last night's leftovers
- soups
- salads – leafy greens such as lettuce with avocado, tomato, cucumber, capsicum, perhaps some cheese, and a good protein source such as bacon, ham, chicken or smoked salmon, topped with an olive oil and balsamic vinegar dressing (try my bacon, feta and avocado salad on page 296)
- meat or fish with vegetables.

Avoid the croutons with your soups or salads, and sugary dressings with your salads.

Dinner

Dinner is pretty easy: meat or fish and plenty of vegetables or salad.

What meat? It doesn't really matter, so that decision is dictated by taste, availability and cost. There's no need to avoid the fatty cuts of meat – the days of trimming all the fat off meat and the skin off chicken are well and truly gone now that we know saturated fat from meat is not at all harmful. I usually cook my meat on the barbecue or pan-fry it in butter.

As far as vegetables go, I would limit starchy vegetables such as potatoes, sweet potatoes and parsnip – and avoid them altogether if I were insulin resistant. Otherwise, pretty much any vegetable is fine. Plenty of colours are a good idea, so a mixture such as spinach, carrots and cauliflower is both colourful and healthy.

We all agree that vegies are great for our heath. The problem is the way we've always cooked them – boiling or steaming – so they finish up soggy and tasteless. Apart from green beans, peas and asparagus, no more boiling or steaming for me. My favourite way of cooking vegies is roasting them. It's easy, low-effort, and very tasty. I add plenty of salt and herbs, such as thyme, oregano, basil, parsley or rosemary, then serve with a bit of butter.

And don't forget the healthy pizza, pasta or rice alternatives on pages 110–11.

Here are some of my favourite dinners:

- baked salmon with soy and sesame (recipe page 298)
- zoodle carbonara (recipe page 297)
- fillet steak with green beans and cauliflower
- lamb backstrap with zucchini and sweet potatoes
- veal scaloppini in a creamy mushroom sauce with cauliflower rice
- pork shoulder with spinach and carrots
- roast beef/lamb/pork/chicken with roast veg.

Dessert

Most desserts are full of sugar, so I tend to avoid them except on special occasions. My fave dessert is berries with full-fat pure cream or full-fat Greek yoghurt. Any combination of strawberries, raspberries, blueberries and blackberries is fine. Berries do have a small amount of carbs so be careful about the volume if you're insulin resistant.

A treat

After dinner, when I'm sitting at my desk (usually) or in front of the TV (rarely), I like a coffee or a green tea, and with that a couple of squares of dark chocolate, at least 70 per cent and preferably 85 per cent cacao. As I noted earlier, dark chocolate is more satiating than milk chocolate, so it's much easier to stop after two squares.

Snacks

With a couple of healthy meals of minimal carbs, healthy fats and adequate protein, you're not likely to get hungry during the day. If you do, however, it's important to avoid the easy snacks often freely available in workplaces or convenience stores, such as flour-based products (muffins and bagels), snack bars (muesli bars), potato chips and confectionery.

My two favourite snacks are nuts and cheese. Nuts are a healthy satiating snack and could be one of or a combination of macadamias, almonds, Brazil nuts, hazelnuts, peanuts and cashews. Avoid overindulging – a handful of nuts goes a long way. Cheese is also a filling and nutritious snack. You could try a hard cheese such as cheddar or one of the soft cheeses such as a brie or camembert.

Unless you're severely limiting carbs, a piece of fruit such as an apple or pear can be an excellent snack, as well as a full-fat yoghurt. You could also try a hard-boiled egg, some dried meat (e.g. biltong), or some chopped vegies (carrots, zucchini, celery) with dips such as hummus, guacamole or cream cheese.

POINTS TO REMEMBER

- We traditionally eat three meals a day, but you should eat when it suits your lifestyle and when you are hungry.
- Try yoghurt with nuts, seeds or berries or eggs with bacon, mushrooms, tomatoes, avocados or smoked salmon for breakfast; soups or salads for lunch; and meat or fish and plenty of vegetables for dinner.
- For snacks avoid processed sugary and starchy foods – nuts and cheese are filling and healthy.

My Top Twenty Real Foods

What I like to eat and know is excellent for our health.

By now you've probably figured out my favourite foods, but here's my list: all tasty, real food, full of nutrients, with no sugar or seed oils.

1. Avocado
2. Eggs
3. Salmon
4. Nuts – macadamias, almonds, walnuts, hazelnuts
5. Butter – grass-fed
6. Full-fat Greek yoghurt
7. Cream
8. Cheese
9. Coconut oil
10. Olive oil
11. Green vegetables – broccoli, beans, zucchini, spinach
12. Cauliflower
13. Grass-fed meat – beef, lamb, pork, chicken
14. Bacon
15. Bone broth
16. Apple cider vinegar
17. Green tea
18. Liver and other organ meats
19. Berries – blueberries, raspberries, strawberries, blackberries
20. Dark chocolate

Don't Blow the Food Budget

You can eat well on a budget.

By now you might be thinking, 'Yeah, Doc, it's all very well to eat all these nutrient-dense real foods, but I can't afford it. Going to Maccas is a lot cheaper.'

Fair call – real food can be a bit more expensive. But how much is your own health and your family's health worth? And how does your grocery bill compare to an enormous medical bill a few years down the track?

Research published in 2016 actually found that diets following the recommendations of the Australian Dietary Guidelines are *cheaper* than current diets, which tend to be less healthy.[1] Depending on the household, the guidelines diet cost 66–99 per cent of the money currently being spent on food and drinks. Australian nutritionist Amanda Lee, the author of the study, said that 'the perception is that healthier foods are more expensive than unhealthy foods. And when you compare the price of selected individual items this might be the case. But when you anchor the cost of what people are actually eating to their total diet, a healthier diet is actually cheaper.'[2]

It's definitely possible to eat healthily on a budget, so let's look at some ways of getting good food within your household budget:

- **Eat at home**: Eating out is expensive, and it's much cheaper to buy your own ingredients and cook at home. Cooking for yourself also gives you the huge bonus of knowing exactly what's going into your meal – no risk of sugars and seed oils sneaking their way in!
- **Plan your meals for the week**: Work out your breakfast, lunch and dinner for each day and make a grocery list for anything not in your pantry. Before the week starts, batch-cook a couple of meals so they're ready to reheat quickly during the week.
- **Use leftovers**: Leftovers are a good option for meals the next day, such as kids' school lunches. Get into the habit of cooking extra so you'll

always have leftovers and make the time spent cooking go further. Depending on how creative you feel, you can turn your leftovers into something else.

- **Don't waste your vegetables**: If you think you're not going to get around to eating those vegetables you bought, freeze them. Alternatively . . .
- **Buy frozen vegetables and berries**: Fresh vegetables and berries can be expensive, especially out of season. Frozen foods are available all year round and are still healthy.
- **Invest in a large freezer**: Buy foods such as meat and vegetables in bulk when on sale and then freeze what you won't use. It's great to know you have things on hand for emergencies without having to go to the shops.
- **Buy cheaper store brands rather than popular labels**: Foods such as frozen vegetables or tinned goods will often be much cheaper if you buy own-brand products rather than a well-known label. Just remember to check the ingredients to avoid added sugar.
- **Get your timing right**: Fresh food markets or farmers' markets often discount foods towards the end of trading hours so they're not left with unsold food. Find out what time prices start to be slashed and do your shopping then.
- **Try cheaper cuts of meat**: Instead of boneless, skinless chicken breasts, buy chicken legs or thighs. Put a budget-friendly pork shoulder or roasting beef in the oven or slow-cooker to feed the whole family with leftovers to spare. It's usually a better deal to buy a whole chicken and to cut it into pieces yourself. Use the carcass to make chicken broth (see recipe page 303).
- **Eat eggs**: Eggs are a great, cheap source of good-quality protein. I eat two or three free-range eggs for breakfast most days.
- **Make your own yoghurt**: It's easy, delicious, healthy and cheap.
- **Buy spices, nuts and seeds in bulk**: This is often an option in health food stores.
- **Make up your own 'muesli'**: I make up a mix of nuts and seeds (no grains) using bulk-purchased product, which I love to eat with yoghurt and berries (see recipe page 293).

- **Grow your own**: Herbs are easy to grow, and some vegetables need very little care – and a surprising number can be grown in pots. If you want your kids to eat vegies, get them involved in planting, watering and harvesting them, and then get them to help in their preparation and cooking.
- **Drink tap water**: In most areas of Australia the tap water is fine for drinking. There's no need to buy bottled water. For added flavour make up a jug with some sliced lemon, lime, cucumber or berries, and add some mint.
- **Shop at discount grocers**: Some will offer healthy organic food for less than mainstream grocery chains.
- **Use coupons and loyalty programs**.

It *is* possible to eat good healthy food without blowing your budget – it just requires planning and good organisation. And once you've given it a go, you'll start to find it becomes second nature – not to mention even quite fun.

POINTS TO REMEMBER
- Eating healthily on a budget is more than possible by using a few simple tricks.

Fast Food Doesn't Necessarily Mean Junk Food

You can order well in fast-food chains if you make the effort.

It's fair to say that increased patronage of fast-food chains has contributed to our poor health. This is because most items sold by these chains are high in sugar (health enemy number 1) or processed carbohydrates, and cooked in vegetable oils (health enemy number 2). Finding healthy options at fast-food chain outlets has always been a problem, but increasingly the chains are including healthier options in their menus in response to public demand – meaning fast food no longer strictly has to be junk food as long as you're savvy.

General guidelines

There are a few general rules of thumb you can apply to almost any fast-food outlet:

- **Stick to meat, cheese, and vegetables**: Try to keep to the basics, and avoid breads, sauces and condiments.
- **Go for grilled, not fried**: A number of fast-food restaurants now offer grilled, broiled or roasted chicken and beef options. Add a side of vegetables and you've got yourself a relatively healthy fast-food meal.
- **Limit the chips**: Hot chips are full of starch and cooked in seed oils – not a good combination! Studies show that eating fries may trigger cravings for more.[1]
- **Avoid the bun**: Some establishments let you order a burger wrapped in lettuce leaves, or you can always remove the bun and eat the insides with a fork. Keep your burger simple, with meat, lettuce and tomato.
- **Choose salad**: Salads remain some of the best low-carb items on fast-food menus. Opt for simpler salads that include meat, such as grilled chicken plus lettuce, tomato and cucumber, and ask for the dressing

on the side. Avoid extras like creamy sauces, croutons, cheeses and tortilla strips. Pick a low-sugar salad dressing like oil and vinegar. You can also opt for no salad dressing if there are no healthy options.

- **Keep away from breadcrumbs**: Chicken wings and other fried items will typically have a coating of wheat flour-based breadcrumbs. If you can, try to order your food with no breadcrumbs. Many chicken wing restaurants offer naked (traditional) chicken wings as an option. If you have no other choice, try to peel off as much of the crumbs as you possibly can.
- **Watch the sauces and dressings**: Sauces and dressings are usually filled with sugar, so avoid sweet-tasting sauces and try to opt for fattier salad dressings. Sometimes you can't avoid either – in some places they'll squirt tomato or barbecue sauce on automatically – so ask for no sauce or sauce on the side when you order.
- **Drink water**: Avoid soft drinks, fruit juices and flavoured milks.
- **Choose breakfast carefully**: Most breakfast items from fast-food restaurants are loaded with carbohydrates – pancakes, muffins, bagels, waffles and biscuits. Some fast-food outlets will have an option with eggs, bacon, mushrooms and tomatoes.

Healthy options at fast-food chains

It's almost always possible to stick with your healthy eating if you keep your wits about you.

McDonald's

Just remove the bun or, better still, ask for a bun-less burger wrapped in lettuce if available. Then add extras such as cheese, bacon, onions, tomato, avocado and mustard. Avoid the French fries, soft drinks, mayonnaise and tomato sauce. Other non-burger options include egg or sausage McMuffins without the bread, and salads.

KFC

KFC has a number of grilled chicken options in flatbread or wraps, including chicken salad, chicken Caesar and BLT 'twisters', which you can eat without the bread/wrap.

Mexican

Most Mexican restaurants will allow you to leave out the tortilla and other high-carb items. This is known as a burrito bowl or 'bare' burrito. A burrito bowl can include meat (pork, beef, chicken), grilled onions, capsicum, cheese, sour cream, lettuce, guacamole and salsa. No bowls? No problem. Unwrap your burrito and eat the contents with a fork. When you're finished, discard the tortilla.

Pizza

Most pizza places offer chicken wings. If it has to be pizza, load up on toppings and eat as little of the crust as possible. Ask for a knife and fork to help you avoid eating the crust.

Subway

Subway is the most popular fast-food sandwich shop worldwide. In recent years, the chain has been offering chopped salads that can be customised with meat (roast beef, chicken, ham, turkey, meatballs, tuna), eggs, or BLT with vegetables of your choice.

Kebabs

These can be extremely low in carbs if you ask for extra salad and eat the meat and salad out of the bread wrap with a fork. Again, avoid the sauces.

Indian

Indian cuisine offers many good options for adventurous healthy eaters. Choose kebabs, curries (without potatoes), meat in creamy sauces (like chicken tikka masala and butter chicken), and tandoori dishes. Skip the rice and the naan bread. Try adding raita (a creamy dip made from plain yoghurt and shredded cucumbers).

Asian

Proceed with caution at Chinese, Japanese, Thai and Vietnamese restaurants. Focus on staying away from options that are battered or taste sweet. Stir-fries or curries made with meat, seafood and low-carb vegetables taste great without the rice. Order crispy duck (ensure it comes without a sweet sauce) or chop suey. If you find shirataki (yam) noodles on a Japanese menu, note that they're very low in carbohydrates.

Chinese

There's wide variation in Chinese food, depending both on where in China the cuisine is from and on where the restaurant is – in some parts of Australia, there's often also an extensive 'Australian' menu. For low-carb Chinese, it's best to avoid or limit: rice (fried and steamed), noodles (including chow mein, lo mein and chow fun), wontons and dumplings (including the deep-fried type), crumbed meats and egg rolls. It's also important to avoid sweet sauces such as sweet and sour, plum, oyster, hoisin and duck sauces. Spicy sauces tend to have sugar in them, so ask about this. Lemon chicken almost always has a lot of sugar. Peking duck and moo shu pork are fine, although you may need to avoid the pancakes and plum sauce on the side if you're trying to limit carbs. Thick soups and sauces are often thickened with cornflour.

For an entrée, try egg drop soup instead of fried wontons or an egg roll. The soup should be clear and thin rather than thickened with cornflour. Instead of prawn, pork, beef or chicken fried rice or noodle dishes, have a sizzling prawn platter, steamed tofu with vegetables, or beef with Chinese mushrooms. If it comes with a sauce, request it be served on the side. Rather than any of the sweet and sour dishes, try stir-fried pork with garlic sauce on the side.

My recommended choices are:

- clear thin soups
- steamed food, including whole steamed fish or steamed tofu with vegetables
- meat and vegetable combinations with thin savoury sauces such as chicken with mushrooms (in many places), moo goo gai pan, Szechuan prawns and curry chicken
- stir-fried dishes
- black bean sauce
- moo shu without the wrappers
- walnut chicken
- egg foo yung (without gravy).

Japanese

The Japanese are among the healthiest people on earth and this is thought to be due to their high intake of fish and seaweed, and relatively low intake of sugar and processed carbohydrates. If cutting back on carbs, limit or avoid the noodles and rice. Healthy options include:

- sashimi
- seaweed salads
- grilled chicken/beef with vegetables (donburi)
- miso soup.

Thai

Healthy Thai options include:

- soups (tom kha gai, Thai coconut chicken soup and coconut-curried cauliflower)
- stir-fries
- salads
- Thai chicken.

Vietnamese

Healthy Vietnamese options include:

- classics such as pho (fragrant soup) and bun cha (grilled pork and noodles), with extra vegies (bean sprouts, cabbage) instead of the noodles
- goi (Vietnamese salad)
- bo la lot (flame-grilled beef wrapped in betel leaf)
- com suon without the rice (com)
- bo bit tet (beef steak)
- bo luc lac (sauteed beef).

POINTS TO REMEMBER
- Foods from fast-food outlets tend to be high in processed carbs and cooked in seed oil.
- Increasingly the big chains are offering healthy alternatives, including grilled rather than fried food.
- It's possible to find healthy options at Asian fast-food outlets by limiting fried foods, sweet sauces, rice and noodles.

Eating Out

It's possible to eat well when eating out,
and will become second nature.

A lot of people say to me, 'You can't eat low-carb real food when you go out to restaurants.' I eat out a lot, having been on the road with sporting teams for up to ten months of the year over the past few years, and throughout all those years of restaurant and hotel meals, I can honestly say I've never been unable to find a healthy low-carb real food option.

It can sometimes be a bit of a challenge, though, so let me share with you some of my tips and tricks.

- **Don't eat the bread**: Many restaurants serve bread while you're waiting for your ordered courses to arrive. Give it a miss.
- **Starters**: Healthy starters include seafood such as oysters, prawns and scallops. Smoked salmon is often available, and there's often an avocado dish. Sashimi is another good option, as are crudités with a dip such as hummus, salsa or vinaigrette. One of my favourite starters is asparagus in a Hollandaise sauce. A charcuterie with ham, prosciutto, salami and other cured meats is another pretty good option. Olives and nuts are good nibbles. And there's nothing better than a home-made soup on a cold winter's evening to start things off.
- **Main course**: Every restaurant has some meat or fish options for main course. Even Italian restaurants with menus that are largely pasta and pizza will always have some meat dishes – my favourite is veal sca-loppini with mushroom and cream sauce. Order your favorite beef, lamb, veal, pork, chicken or fish dish, and just be careful about sauces, which as we know can be full of hidden sugars. Béarnaise sauce, which is made from egg yolks and butter, is good to have with steak, while creamy sauces go well with veal. If you don't like the look of the sauce on the menu just ask for the meat without the sauce, or see if they have a healthier sauce. Asking for the sauce to be served on the side instead

of over the meat gives you the option of leaving it out if you don't want to eat it. I'll often ask for some extra butter and place that on the meat, which is especially nice with steak. Herb butter and garlic butter are good alternatives.

- **Sides**: Some restaurants will give you a choice of sides, which makes it easy – there is usually some sort of green veg or cauliflower or carrot option. Always ask if vegies are included with the meal. The standard vegies served with most meat and fish dishes in Australia are a green vegetable and some sort of potato dish, mashed or chips usually. I simply ask the waiter to hold off on the potatoes and give me extra vegies instead. Some of them might look at you a bit strangely (I'm used to that anyway!), but there's rarely a problem with that request.

- **Salads**: Salads are generally healthy, but the main challenge is always the dressing. Ask for an olive oil and vinegar dressing on the side and drizzle the oil liberally.

- **Drinks**: Water (still or sparkling), tea and coffee are usually available. If you're drinking something alcoholic, stick with red or dry white wine, champagne or spirits with soda water as a mixer.

- **Desserts**: It's probably best to give the dessert menu a miss unless they have some berries and cream. The cheese platter is a good option if you're still hungry.

- **Buffet restaurants**: The all-you-can-eat buffet can be a problem – somehow it's harder to resist foods when they're sitting right in front of you than when they have to be ordered from a menu, and we all like getting value for money! So discipline is required when you head to the buffet. Use a smaller plate if possible, and try not to return for seconds – remember portion sizes. The good thing about buffets is there is usually plenty of choice, including healthy options – you just have to find them. Focus on the healthy food – the salad bar, carvery, seafood spreads and vegetable platters. And you can usually find some healthy fats, such as olive oil, butter, sour cream and cheese to add to your plate.

- **Breakfasts**: Eating out at breakfast (or brunch) presents a few challenges. For cold options, avoid the breakfast cereals and be careful about the Bircher muesli or granola if you're watching your grain intake. With luck, there'll be a full-fat Greek yoghurt option rather than the sugar-filled fruit yoghurts. Eggs are a good choice, with sides of bacon, mushrooms, tomatoes, smoked salmon or avocado. Ask for the eggs without toast if you're cutting back on grains, or request sourdough or wholegrain toast if not. Avoid the fruit juices and go with water, tea or coffee.

POINTS TO REMEMBER

- It isn't difficult to eat healthy, nutritious food when you eat out.
- Be careful what you order and request healthy alternatives.
- Avoid too much bread, sugary sauces and dressings, starchy vegetables, desserts and soft drinks.

Reading Food Labels

Food labels aren't as helpful as they should be,
but here are some tips.

In an ideal world you wouldn't actually need this section, because most real foods (meat, fish, vegetables, fruit, water) don't have food labels on them. I know . . . life isn't that simple.

All packaged or processed foods have lists of ingredients and a nutrition panel on the back or side of the packet, and this is the information that will help you make the best purchase. Get into the habit of taking a look at the label before you put anything in your trolley, and comparing similar products or brands to find out which is the healthiest. Soon enough you'll know which are the ones to choose and to avoid.

List of ingredients

Ingredients are listed in descending order of use by weight from most to least, so pay particular attention to the first three or four ingredients.

There are two things that get me worried:

1. **A long list of ingredients:** More ingredients are a sign of ultra-processed food, and this can't be healthy. Avoid foods with more than six to eight items on the ingredients list.
2. **Sugar first or second on the list:** If sugar (or one of the alternative names for sugar listed on page 312) is one of the first two ingredients, there's probably too much sugar in it. Be aware that sometimes manu-facturers split up sugar into dextrose, high-fructose corn syrup, cane crystals and so on, so that none of them are the first ingredient – even though if you added them up, they would be. Sneaky!

Nutrition panels

The key elements of the nutrition panels are the carbohydrate and sugar content. I'm not too fussed about the other components, myself.

Nutrition Information (AVERAGE) Servings per package - 6 Serving size - 35g (1 metric cup†)	quantity per serving	% daily intake ▲ per serving	per serve with 1/2 cup skim milk	quantity per 100g
ENERGY	540 kJ	6%	740 kJ	1550 kJ
PROTEIN	2.7 g	5%	7.4 g	7.7 g
FAT, TOTAL	0.1 g	0.1%	0.2 g	0.2 g
- SATURATED	<0.1 g	0.1%	0.2 g	0.1 g
CARBOHYDRATE	28.5 g	9%	34.9 g	81.3 g
- SUGARS	2.7 g	3%	9.2 g	7.7 g
DIETARY FIBRE	1.4 g	5%	1.4 g	4.1 g
SODIUM	183 mg	8%	240 mg	525 mg
		%RDI*		
THIAMIN (VIT B1)	0.28 mg	25%	0.33 mg	0.79 mg
RIBOFLAVIN (VIT B2)	0.42 mg	25%	0.68 mg	1.21 mg
NIACIN	2.5 mg	25%	2.6 mg	7.1 mg
VITAMIN C	6.0 mg	15%	7.3 mg	17.1 mg
FOLATE	100 µg	50%	106 µg	285 µg
IRON	3.0 mg	25%	3.1 mg	8.6 mg
ZINC	1.8 mg	15%	2.3 mg	5.1 mg

† Cup measurement is approximate and is only to be used as a guide. If you have any specific dietary requirements please weigh your serving.
▲ Percentage daily intakes are based on an average adult diet of 8700kJ.
* Percentage Recommended Dietary Intake (Aust/NZ)

- **Servings per package and average serving size**: The serving size could seem very small, so if you're likely to eat more than that, make sure you factor that in when working out how much sugar there is. The food companies themselves are free to choose the serving sizes, which explains why they're so unpredictable and sometimes downright odd.
- **Nutrient columns – per serve and per 100 g**: Use the per 100 g column to determine what percentage of each item. A product with 20 g sugar per 100 g will be 20 per cent or one-fifth sugar.
- **Energy**: The number of kilojoules of energy contained in the food. One calorie = approximately 4 kilojoules.
- **Protein**: This isn't that important given most Australians get enough protein.

- **Fat – total and saturated**: I find this pretty useless, as it doesn't tell you the important thing – how much monounsaturated, polyunsaturated, omega-3 and omega-6 there is.
- **Carbohydrates and sugar**: As a rule, I recommend sticking to foods with no more than 3–5 g of sugar per 100 g – and certainly less than 10 g per 100 g.
- **Fibre**: The nutrition information panel does not need to include fibre unless a nutrition claim is made on the label about fibre, sugar or carbohydrate – 'high in fibre', say, or 'low in sugar'. Around 3 g per 100 g is a significant amount of fibre.
- **Sodium**: Be aware that sodium is often given in milligrams (mg) rather than grams. To calculate the percentage of sodium in this case, you have to divide by 1000 first. Remember, I suggested a total daily intake of 3200–4800 mg per day.

Nutrition claims

What do they mean and are they true?

- **'Low fat'**: To be in this category, a product must have 3 grams of fat or less per 100 grams – but check the label, because it's probably high in sugar instead.
- **'Fat free' or 'no fat'**: To be in this category, a food product must have 0.15 grams fat or less per 100 grams food. Again, check for sugar.
- **'Lite' or 'light'**: Always check the nutrition information panel on these foods because 'lite' may mean the food is light in colour or taste or something else, but as a result is heavy in sugar.
- **'No added sugar'**: This food has no 'added' sugar but may still be high in natural sugar and high-GI, so check the sugar content on the nutrition information panel.
- **'Low joule' or 'diet'**: It's low in sugar and/or fat and may be artificially sweetened.
- **'No added salt'**: It has no 'added' salt but may still be high in natural salt, so if you're worried, check the sodium content on the nutrition information panel.
- **'Salt reduced'**: This food has 25 per cent less salt than a similar product, but it doesn't automatically mean it's low in sodium.

- **'Low salt' or 'low sodium'**: The food must have less than 120 milligrams of sodium per 100 grams.
- **'High fibre'**: It must have more than 3 grams of fibre per 100 grams.
- **'Baked not fried'**: Not necessarily lower in fat or energy, so check the label if that bothers you.
- **'Cholesterol free'**: This only makes sense for animal products. It could still be high in fat or energy, if you're worried about those things.
- **'Natural' or 'organic'**: May have the same amount of sugars, fats or energy as regular varieties.
- **'Wholegrain'**: There's no definition or standard for labelling for percentage of wholegrains.
- **'Gluten-free'**: There is no detectable level of gluten.

Healthy food ratings

A number of ratings have been produced over the years to assist the consumer in choosing healthy food. Unfortunately, as they're mainly based on the outdated guidelines to 'avoid saturated fat and cholesterol, and eat lots of carbs', they're often misleading. The main rating system at the moment is the Health Star Rating.

Health Star Rating

This front-of-pack labelling scheme was developed for use in Australia and New Zealand, ostensibly to 'provide convenient, relevant and readily understood nutrition information and/or guidance on packaged food to assist consumers to make informed food purchases and healthier eating choices'.[1] Star ratings are based on lower energy, saturated fat, sodium and (to some extent) sugar content, and may also reflect higher dietary fibre, protein, fruit, vegetable, legume and nut content. There are different criteria for different food groups.

Unfortunately, the ratings are invalidated for three reasons:

1. They don't account properly for sugar.
2. They penalise healthy fats.
3. They penalise salt.

As a result they produce numerous anomalies. Plain milk gets four stars out of five, while a liquid breakfast and low-fat strawberry milk get four and a half stars! Milo, which is just under half sugar, gets four and half stars. Nutri-Grain, which is more than a quarter sugar, gets four stars. Commercial fruit juice gets between four and five stars and a supermarket brand's beer-battered frozen steakhouse chips four stars. Packaged smoked salmon, however, only manages three and a half stars, while plain natural Greek yoghurt rates a measly one and a half.

Perhaps this is not so surprising when you discover that:

1. The food industry sits on the Health Star Rating advisory panel (members include the Australian Food and Grocery Council and major supermarkets).
2. The system isn't mandatory.
3. It's based on nutrients, not whole foods.
4. It gives no indication of how much processing a food has gone through.

Dr Kieron Rooney, a senior lecturer in the Faculty of Health Sciences at the University of Sydney, described the rating as 'not much more than a marketing tool for industry'; while journalist and author Peter FitzSimons – who lost 45 kilograms when he gave up sugar – writes, 'Any health star system that doesn't identify added sugar as the prime culprit is not serious.'[2]

POINTS TO REMEMBER
- Beware foods with a long list of ingredients, and avoid foods where sugar (by any name) is first or second on the list.
- 'Low fat' usually means high-sugar.
- The Health Star Ratings are flawed due their over-emphasis on saturated fat and under-emphasis on sugar.

Supplements

Most of us don't need supplements if we eat real food.

The supplement business is huge and worth billions of dollars a year. I am going to start this chapter by stating up front: I don't take any supplements myself. I'm not saying no one should, I just feel that I can get all the nutrients I need from a diet full of real foods that avoids sugar, processed foods and vegetable oils.

Let's have a closer look at some of the supplements for which there's some scientific evidence they might work.

Protein shakes

Protein shakes based on protein powders are very popular among those wishing to bulk up or aid recovery after a workout, and have been shown to be effective in gaining muscle bulk (in conjunction with resistance exercise), weight loss and improved recovery.[1] Most of the popular supplements on the market are based on whey or casein, by-products of the cheese-making process. Whey protein is low in lactose, easily digestible and contains all the essential amino acids. Casein (milk protein) is more slowly digested and takes longer for the body to assimilate. Proteins from plants such as brown rice, pea and soy are used by vegans.

The majority of the popular commercial powders are whey-based and contain 70–80 per cent protein, 5–12 per cent carbs and less than 10 per cent fat. Protein powders can be:

- **Protein concentrate**: This is the most typical form of protein powder. Whey concentrate is 70–80 per cent protein by weight.
- **Protein isolate**: This starts as a concentrate but then undergoes an isolation process to remove the carbohydrates and fat. It therefore has a higher protein content than standard protein concentrates. For whey, this is usually 90–93 per cent protein by weight.
- **Protein hydrolysate**: The manufacturing process uses either heat or

mild acid to break down the amino acids and produce a hydrolysate. The result is digested faster and 90–95 per cent protein.

Protein powders are mixed with milk (dairy or nut milk) or water, fruits (berries, avocado), vegetables, chocolate, peanut butter and anything else you can think of. Try to stick to the pure powders, and avoid those containing vegetable oils and sugars.

BCAAs

Amino acids are simple compounds that are the building blocks of protein and muscle. Three of the 20 found in the human body help increase protein synthesis within muscle. These three – leucine, isoleucine and valine – are collectively known as the branched-chain amino acids or BCAAs.

Supplements containing BCAAs are popular alternatives to protein powders, but BCAAs seem to have no particular advantage over whole protein powders (such as whey) or food sources of protein (such as eggs). It appears that for full muscle growth we need a sufficient supply of the whole complement of amino acids.

Vitamins

Over the years, various vitamins have been the flavour of the month. At various times we've convinced ourselves of the health value of vitamins C, A and B, but there's little evidence to support supplementing with these.

What about a multivitamin tablet once a day? This sounds reasonably attractive – you're covering lots of different vitamins (and minerals if it's a combined vitamin/mineral supplement) and you're not going to overdose on any one vitamin. The corollary to that is that there's so little of each of the vitamins in a multivitamin tablet that there's probably no point. Most of it will probably be excreted as expensive wee.

The other concern with these multivitamin tablets and any other supplements is that all sorts of additives are included, such as soy, gluten, corn, hydrogenated oils, preservatives, GMOs, colourings/dyes, and binders like magnesium stearate. If you take a supplement, look for one that's organic, based on whole foods, and either raw or low-temperature heated. Also make sure it contains minerals, which are important for vitamin absorption.

There are two specific vitamins that I would like to discuss in some detail. One is vitamin D (see page 237) and the second is the little-known vitamin K2.

Vitamin K2 is an important vitamin but seems to have flown under the radar. There's good evidence that it's beneficial for cardiovascular health and may help reduce the risk of cancer.[2] It also seems to work well in combination with vitamin D in getting calcium into bones.[3] Fortunately, vitamin K2 is found in many of the nutrient-dense real foods I've been advocating, including bacon, butter from grass-fed cows, chicken, egg yolks, grass-fed beef, hard cheese, liver, pastured pork, prosciutto and salami. Many health organisations promote vegetables as the best source of vitamin K, but they contain vitamin K1 which the body then needs to convert to K2.

Calcium

For many years, calcium supplements were recommended for those at risk of deficiency (post-menopausal women, female athletes and those who avoid dairy), and even perfectly healthy people. But more recent research indicates that calcium supplements are not well absorbed, and they're no longer recommended for post-menopausal women.[4]

Some studies actually showed that calcium supplements were associated with a higher risk of fractures and possibly cardiovascular disease. A meta-analysis of studies involving more than 12 000 participants found that calcium supplementation increases the risk of heart attack by 31 per cent, stroke by 20 per cent and death from all causes by 9 per cent.[5]

Calcium from food sources is more efficiently absorbed by the body. The main dietary source of calcium is dairy, but even if you're dairy intolerant, you can obtain calcium from many other foods, such as bone broth, fish with bones (tinned salmon and sardines), nuts (almonds, hazelnuts, pistachios), vegetables (broccoli, kale), figs, beans, seaweeds, sesame seeds and tofu.

Magnesium

Magnesium is the current 'flavour of the month' supplement. We don't actually need much magnesium to function well, but magnesium deficiency is said to be widespread. Magnesium deficiency has been linked with various conditions, such as high blood pressure, migraine, muscle cramps and depression.

Magnesium deficiency does seem to be common and there are several explanations. They include soil depletion leading to lower magnesium levels in crops, malabsorption of magnesium in the gut due to digestive disorders, and medications such as antibiotics affecting magnesium absorption in the gut.

The body loses magnesium stores through daily functions such as muscle movement, heartbeat and hormone production. Although we only need small amounts, it must be replaced regularly to prevent deficiency. Magnesium is found in green leafy vegetables, avocados, bananas, melons, legumes, nuts, seeds and certain whole grains.

Magnesium citrate, chelate and chloride supplement forms are absorbed better than magnesium oxide and sulfate supplements.

Fish oil

Fish oil is an effective way of obtaining healthy omega-3 fats. About 30 per cent of fish oil is omega-3 fats, and the remaining 70 per cent is other fats. The omega-3s in fish oil, eicosapentaenoic acid (EPA) and docosahexaenoic acid (DHA), have greater health benefits than the alpha-linolenic acid (ALA) found in some plant sources.

Studies initially found that fish oil was beneficial for heart disease, particularly over the short term, but most evidence now suggests that it neither prevents nor improves heart disease.[6] The story is similar for metabolic syndrome and cancer.

Recently, attention has been drawn to the quality of over-the-counter fish oil supplements. DHA and EPA can oxidise with exposure to light, oxygen and heat. Oxidised fats have been linked to a number of health issues, including atherosclerosis.

Whole foods are always better than supplements. While fish oil may not protect you, most studies show that eating fish can lower the risk of heart disease and early death.[7] The best way to ensure adequate intake of quality omega-3 fats is to eat two meals of cold-water oily fish or shellfish each week.

If for some reason you don't eat fish, choose a supplement with 300–500 mg EPA and DHA per 1000 mg of fish oil. To help absorb the omega-3 fatty acids, take your fish oil supplement with a meal that contains fat.

Turmeric

If I *was* going to take one supplement I would probably go for turmeric, the spice that gives curry its yellow colour. It's been used in India for thousands of years as a spice and medicinal herb. The active compounds in turmeric are called curcuminoids, the most important of which is curcumin.

Curcumin is an antioxidant with anti-inflammatory effects.[8] The curcumin content of turmeric powder is very low (about 3 per cent by weight), and most of the studies have used turmeric extracts with much higher percentages of curcumin that would be very difficult to manage just by adding turmeric powder to your foods. If you want to experience the full effects, you need to take an extract with significant amounts of curcumin.

Unfortunately, curcumin is poorly absorbed into the bloodstream, but piperine, a natural substance in black pepper, enhances absorption by 2000 per cent.[9] You can either take a combined curcumin and piperine supplement or take a curcumin supplement with ¼ teaspoon black pepper.

Other supplements such as probiotics and prebiotics, as well as Vitamin D and iron, are covered elsewhere in this book.

POINTS TO REMEMBER
- It's probably better to obtain all your necessary nutrients from real foods rather than supplements. There's not much evidence to support taking a daily multivitamin tablet.
- Vitamin K2 is beneficial to the cardiovascular system and can be found in foods such as bacon, butter from grass-fed cows, chicken, egg yolks, grass-fed beef, hard cheese, liver, pastured pork, prosciutto and salami.
- There's some evidence to support taking fish oil and turmeric, but not enough to convince me to take supplements.

Sweeteners

It's best to avoid all sweeteners, whether or not they claim to be natural.

While a healthy diet should ideally emphasise real, whole foods, some people enjoy using low-carb sweeteners. In 2016 the market for food sweeteners was valued at USD $85 billion. It is estimated to reach nearly USD $118 billion by 2022.[1]

Each week, more than a quarter of Australians use sweeteners in both carbonated soft drinks and confectionery. Other foods with sweeteners include flavoured yoghurts, table-top sweeteners, cordials, ice cream, jams, flavoured milk, fruit drinks, jelly or milk-based puddings, canned fruit and toppings.

Their main advantage is that, unlike sugars, they don't contain any calories. These sweeteners are all hundreds of times sweeter than sugar. That all sounds good so far – all the benefits of sugar without the problems, right?

Unfortunately, it's not that simple. Sweeteners have been linked with a number of health problems. In one study, people who consumed artificially sweetened soft drinks daily were about three times more likely than people who consumed sugar-sweetened beverages to develop stroke or dementia. However, the quality of this research has been questioned.[2] Others have suggested that type 2 diabetes is more prevalent in those who regularly consumed artificially sweetened soft drinks.[3]

A 14-year French study examined the type 2 diabetes risk in 60 000 women, comparing those who consumed artificially sweetened drinks with those who drank sugar-sweetened beverages. They found that the risk of developing type 2 diabetes was twice as high in the women drinking high levels of artificially sweetened beverages than those consuming similar amounts of sugar-sweetened beverages.[4]

Another study found a correlation between consuming artificially sweetened drinks and health markers related to metabolic syndrome, such as weight, waist-to-hip ratio, fasting blood glucose, haemoglobin A1c (another blood glucose indicator) and glucose tolerance test.[5] A US study found a similar correlation between daily consumption of diet drinks and the risk of metabolic syndrome (36 per cent greater than non-drinkers of diet soft drinks) and of type 2 diabetes (67 per cent greater).[6] And finally, a review of 30 trials involving more than 400 000 subjects concluded that regularly drinking artificial sweeteners could be linked with a higher body mass index (BMI) and risk of diabetes, heart disease or stroke.[7] The same review also indicated that artificial sweeteners were not an effective tool in weight loss.

It is thought that the negative health effects may be due to alterations in the composition and function of the gut microbiome. A human trial found an association between consumption of artificial sweeteners, gut bacteria composition and glucose intolerance.[8]

Some people using large amounts of sweeteners suffer side effects such as headaches, stomach upsets and cravings for sweet foods.

Types of sweetener

Sweeteners can be divided into three groups:

1. sugar alcohols (erythritol, xylitol)
2. artificial sweeteners (aspartame, sucralose)
3. natural sweeteners (stevia).

Characteristics of some common sweeteners

Sweetener	GI	Type	Net carbs (g per 100 g)	Calories (per 100 g)
Erythritol	0	Sugar alcohol	5	20
Xylitol	13	Sugar alcohol	60	240
Maltitol	36	Sugar alcohol	67	270
Sucralose	0–80	Artificial	0	0
Aspartame	0	Artificial	85	352
Saccharin	Variable	Artificial	94	364
Table sugar	63	Processed	100	387
Stevia	0	Natural	5	20
Inulin	0	Natural	1	150
Monk fruit	0	Natural	0–25	0–100
Tagatose	3	Natural	35	150

Sugar alcohols

This name can be a bit confusing as they're not sugar and contain no alcohol! Sugar alcohols are derived from fruits and vegetables through industrial processing, although they're marketed as 'natural products'.

Erythritol

Erythritol is a sugar alcohol produced by fermenting the naturally occurring sugars in corn. It tastes almost exactly like sugar and has no effect on blood sugar or insulin levels. Long-term animal studies have found no evidence that it could be linked to cancer.

Xylitol

Xylitol is a sugar alcohol widely used as a sweetener in chewing gum, toothpaste, and other sugar-free products. It contains significant amounts of carbohydrate, but the body doesn't metabolise them into glucose, which means xylitol has a GI of only 7 and hardly affects blood sugar levels. Several studies show that it can improve dental health by reducing the risk of tooth decay and cavities.[9] It also increases absorption of calcium, which can help protect against osteoporosis.[10]

Eating too much xylitol can cause gas, bloating and diarrhoea. It's also highly toxic to dogs, so keep it out of reach or out of the house altogether.

Other sugar alcohols

Many other sugar alcohols are used in food, but most of these should be avoided because they increase blood sugar levels – including sorbitol, lacitol, glycerol and isomalt.

Artificial sweeteners

The only artificial sweeteners permitted by Food Standards Australia New Zealand are acesulfame potassium or Ace-K, aspartame (aspartic acid and phenylalanine), thaumatin, saccharin, cyclamate and sucralose. Of these aspartame, sucralose and acesulfame are the most commonly used. These artificial sweeteners have been the centre of controversy for many years. Aspartame has been linked to a number of negative health effects, although there's no convincing proof.

Artificial sweetener (additive number)	Sweetness (table sugar = 1)	Top 5 uses
Acesulfame-K (950)	200	Carbonated soft drinks, flavoured yoghurts/mousses, cordials/fruit drinks, confectionery, flavoured milks
Aspartame (951)	180	Carbonated soft drinks, table-top sweeteners, sports, energy and weight management products, flavoured yoghurts/mousses, confectionery
Cyclamate (952)	30	Cordials/fruit drinks, carbonated soft drinks, table-top sweeteners, jellies/milk-based puddings, other desserts/breakfasts
Saccharin (954)	300	Table-top sweeteners, cordials/fruit drinks, carbonated soft drinks, other desserts/breakfasts, jellies/milk-based puddings
Sucralose (955)	600	Carbonated soft drinks, flavoured yoghurts/mousses, cordials/fruit drinks, table-top sweeteners, sports, energy and weight management products

Aspartame

The main concern with aspartame has been a possible link to blood cancers. This has been clearly shown in mice, but the evidence in humans is not as convincing.[11] No cancer risk was detected in recent short- and medium-term trials. The only human trial to show an increased risk was after 18 years.[12]

Sucralose

There have been similar concerns about a possible link between sucralose and cancer. One long-term animal study showed it can cause leukaemia, but no reliable human trials have been completed.[13]

As long as sucralose is used in its liquid rather than powdered form, it has no effect on blood glucose. It's frequently used in baking in combination with less sweet 'bulking' sugar substitutes (such as erythritol).

Table-top sweeteners

The most popular table-top sweetener in Australia is Equal, which consists of dextrose (i.e. glucose) with maltodextrin, aspartame and acesulfame. Other table-top sweeteners in common use are Splenda (sucralose), Sucaryl (cyclamate), Sugarine (saccharin) and Hermesetas (acesulfame).

Diet soft drinks

The diet soft drinks such as Diet Coke, Coke Zero and Pepsi Max are the main users of artificial sweeteners, primarily aspartame and acesulfame. Pepsi Max changed to sucralose a couple of years ago, but had to return to aspartame after an outcry from consumers.

Sweetener content of popular full-strength and diet colas in Australia

Drink	Sweetener	Component (per 100 ml)				
		Caffeine (mg)	Energy (calories)	Carbs (g)	Sugars (g)	Sodium (mg)
Diet Coke	Aspartame, acesulfame	12.8	0.4	0.1	0	15
Coke Zero	Aspartame, acesulfame	9.6	0.3	0.1	0	11
Coke No Sugar	Aspartame, acesulfame	9.6	0.3	0.1	0	4.2
Coke	Cane sugar	9.7	39.4	11	11	12.7
Pepsi	Cane sugar	11	42.3	11.5	11.5	8.5
Pepsi Max	Aspartame, acesulfame	10.3	0	0	0	10

Natural sweeteners

Popular natural sweeteners include stevia and inulin.

Stevia

Stevia is a natural sweetener that is extracted from the leaves of a South American plant known scientifically as *Stevia rebaudiana*.

There are three principal forms of stevia: powdered stevia extract, stevia liquid extract and whole leaf stevia. While the two extracts originate in nature, they also go through an industrial process. In contrast, the pure leaf form of stevia is probably the most natural sweetener available as it is literally just the leaves of the stevia plant. The stevia extracts are incredibly sweet, but the whole leaf stevia has a more subtle sweetness and a slightly bitter aftertaste. Liquid stevia is recommended over powdered stevia as it is the purer extract.

Stevia has a GI of zero and won't raise blood sugar levels. It has been shown to reduce triglyceride levels.[14]

Inulin

Not to be confused with insulin, inulin is a sweetener extracted largely from chicory root. It's often used mixed with other sweeteners. It can caramelise like sugar and has no aftertaste, but too much of it can have a laxative effect.

Not as bad as sugar but . . .

Several natural sweeteners are popular with people who are concerned about their health, including coconut sugar, honey, maple syrup and molasses. While these may contain a few more nutrients than regular sugar, they're metabolised in exactly the same way and cause the same insulin spike. They are, however, slightly 'less bad' than regular sugar.

Coconut sugar

Coconut sugar contains a small amount of fibre and nutrients, but is still high in fructose, and should be eaten in moderation.

Honey

Honey is a thick, golden liquid produced by honeybees that contains trace amounts of vitamins and minerals, as well as an abundance of beneficial antioxidants. As mentioned previously, eating honey for eight weeks significantly lowered 'bad' LDL cholesterol and blood triglycerides in individuals with diabetes and increased 'good' HDL cholesterol.[15] However, in the same study, the blood sugar marker HbA1c was increased. Another study found that eating honey decreased levels of C-reactive protein (CRP), which is a measure of inflammation.[16]

These studies suggest that honey has slightly less harmful effects on blood sugar levels and metabolism than regular sugar. That said, even though honey has some positive health benefits, it is still sugar and should be used sparingly if at all.

Maple syrup

Maple syrup is a thick, sugary liquid made by cooking down the sap of maple trees. It has a high mineral content and at least 24 different types of antioxidant. It is, however, very high in sugar.

Molasses

Molasses is a sweet, brown liquid with a thick, syrup-like consistency made from boiling down sugar cane or sugar beet juice. It contains some vitamins and minerals, as well as several antioxidants, but it's still high in sugar and should be eaten sparingly.

Sweeteners to avoid

Some sugar substitutes should be avoided at all costs.

Agave nectar

Agave nectar, which is produced by the agave plant, is often marketed as a healthy alternative to sugar, but it is 85 per cent fructose, which makes it probably one of the unhealthiest sweeteners on the market.

High-fructose corn syrup

High-fructose corn syrup (HFCS) is a sweetener made from corn syrup and commonly used, especially in the United States, to sweeten processed foods and soft drinks. Its usual composition is 45 per cent sucrose and 55 per cent glucose, which makes it very similar to table sugar. It should be avoided at all costs. Keep an eye out for 'fructose syrup' – it's the same thing.

What I recommend

I recommend avoiding sweeteners in soft drinks. Why? First, I have some concerns about the safety of the artificial sweeteners such as aspartame, and I think it's better to be safe than sorry. Secondly, they don't appear to help with weight loss, which is the main reason for their use. Thirdly, they maintain our addiction to sweetness. I think it's really important to try to reduce that reliance on sweetness, so water and milk still win easily for me as far as cold drinks go.

If I wanted to use a sweetener at all, for example in cooking, I would use stevia or erythritol.

POINTS TO REMEMBER

- Sweeteners are commonly used in diet soft drinks and confectionery. They don't provide any calories and are hundreds of times sweeter than sugar.
- There are three types of sweetener: artificial sweeteners (aspartame, sucralose, etc.), sugar alcohols (erythritol, xylitol) and natural sweeteners (stevia, inulin).
- There are some health concerns about using the artificial sweeteners, and they maintain our addiction to sweetness, which we need to reduce.

Gluten and Other Allergies

It's not your imagination: food sensitivities are real and on the rise.

Food sensitivities seem to be becoming more frequent. Let's have a close look at some of the more common ones.

Gluten

Gluten. One of the most talked about words in nutrition. Is it all a big con or is seemingly every second person actually gluten-sensitive? As usual, the answer lies somewhere in the middle, so let's try to sort fact from fiction.

When I was at medical school back in the 1970s, we learnt about coeliac disease (CD), an autoimmune condition where the body attacks the intestines in response to the gluten protein in wheat and other foods. CD causes mainly abdominal symptoms (discomfort and bloating) and can be detected with a blood test. Back then, people with CD were put on a gluten-free diet and that was the end of it.

The incidence of coeliac disease has indeed increased over the past few decades, but it's still relatively uncommon. More recently, we've started to see people with similar symptoms to CD, or sometimes non-bowel symptoms, who test negative to CD yet respond very well to a gluten-free diet. These people have been diagnosed with gluten sensitivity, and a whole industry has sprung up around gluten-free foods.

Gluten is a group of proteins found in wheat, barley, rye, oats and products made from these. Gluten, which means 'glue' in Latin, gives elasticity to dough, allowing it to rise, and is responsible for the chewy texture of bread and other products.

Wheat contains hundreds of different proteins. CD is characterised by an immune response to one specific protein and a specific enzyme, but we now know that people can (and do) react to several other components of wheat. There's pretty good evidence that many of us are sensitive to one of the wheat proteins, a condition lumped under the term 'gluten sensitivity'. Given the variety of proteins, it would probably be more correct to use a term like 'wheat sensitivity'. Whatever we call it, it responds well to a wheat-free diet.

It's important to remember that gluten sensitivity (and CD) does not necessarily present only as gut symptoms, but can affect nearly every tissue in the body.[1] Because of this and the inability to make a diagnosis on the basis of a simple test, the only way to determine if you have the condition is to trial a wheat-free diet.

Researchers at Monash University in Melbourne believe that rather than gluten being the main culprit in gastrointestinal disorders, it is fructans, a type of sugar chain found in wheat, barley and rye, as well as onions, garlic, chickpeas, cabbage, and artichokes, that are the problem. Wheat products (bread, pasta etc.) and onions seem to be the major problems. They suggest that this may be why changing to a gluten-free diet may lead to some, but not total, improvement in symptoms.[2]

What to do if you're gluten sensitive

I'm not crazy about the large numbers of gluten-free products. I'd prefer to simply avoid grains, which aren't particularly healthy anyway. In fact, when compared with other foods like organ meats, fish, meats, vegetables and fruits, whole grains are at the bottom of the list. And refined grains (like wheat flour) are even lower. Replacing grains with real foods that have nutritional value is preferable to eating highly processed gluten-free products.

If you suspect you may be gluten sensitive, see your GP and, based on their advice, consider putting yourself on a wheat-free diet for 60 days to see what effect that has on your symptoms. After 60 days you can 'challenge' yourself with a couple of slices of bread and see what happens.

Many people who are intolerant of gluten are also intolerant of other proteins found in foods like dairy, eggs and, unfortunately, coffee. Studies have shown that about 50 per cent of people with CD show intolerance to casein, a protein in milk.[3] This may explain why up to 30 per cent of CD patients continue to experience symptoms after adopting a gluten-free diet. For this reason, some recommend a completely grain- and dairy-free diet during the trial period.

If you have CD, it's likely that your gut lining is damaged and you'll need to heal it. To do this you should initially avoid sugars, soy products, processed foods and vegetable oils, all of which increase inflammation in the gut.

FODMAPs

Gluten is not the only sensitivity associated with bowel symptoms. A certain percentage of people with irritable bowel syndrome (IBS), which causes symptoms such abdominal pain, bloating and diarrhoea, are sensitive to a group of carbohydrates known as FODMAPs. This is an acronym for the carbohydrates involved:

> Fermentable – meaning they're broken down (fermented) by bacteria in the large intestine.
> Oligosaccharides – 'oligo' means 'few' and 'saccharide' means sugar. These are sugars longer than disaccharides and shorter than polysaccharides.
> Disaccharides – double sugars.
> Monosaccharides – single sugars.
> and Polyols – sugar alcohols (but they don't lead to intoxication!).

As with gluten sensitivity, there's no one simple test to diagnose FODMAP sensitivity. People tend not to be sensitive to all of these substances, so it's a matter of removing the FODMAPs from your diet and seeing what effect that has.

Foods that contain FODMAPs include:

- vegetables: asparagus, onions, garlic, legumes, beetroot, celery, corn
- fruit: apples, pears, mangoes, watermelon, nectarines, peaches, plums
- dairy: cow's milk, yoghurt, soft cheese, cream, custard, ice cream
- grains: rye- and wheat-containing breads, wheat-based cereals with dried fruit, wheat pasta.

Obviously removing all these foods is very restrictive, but a low-FODMAP diet is not designed to be permanent. It's really a type of elimination diet; it's highly restrictive for several weeks, before foods are slowly reintroduced to determine what causes symptoms. There's a particular order for reintroducing foods efficiently to determine a particular sensitivity, so you'll need to do some research if you want to go down this road.

Food allergies and intolerances

Given the number of chemicals contained in what we currently refer to as 'food', it shouldn't be a great surprise that food allergies and intolerances are on the increase. Australia leads the world in the incidence of proven food allergies in young children over five years of age, with an incidence of around 10 per cent.[4]

A food *allergy* is an immune response to a food that occurs whenever that food is eaten and generates adverse health effects. The immune system produces antibodies to substances in these foods and inflammatory substances called cytokines that can result in an acute, and sometimes life-threatening, allergic response, such as anaphylactic shock.

Food *intolerances*, on the other hand, are typically associated with enzymatic deficiencies, malabsorption or sensitivity to certain food components such as gluten or histamine. They can cause a wide variety of gastrointestinal and inflammatory symptoms, but aren't life-threatening.

Recent research seems to indicate that changes in the normal human microbiome can be a factor in the development of food allergies and intolerances.[5] In some cases, restoring balance to the gut microbiome can alleviate these allergies and intolerances, and potentially restore tolerance to the foods that trigger them.

Insufficient exposure to microorganisms in early childhood is thought to alter the gut microbiome, suppress the normal development of the immune system and increase susceptibility to allergic disease. Researchers have found clear differences in the microbiomes of food-allergic and non-allergic people. The lack of exposure results from a number of factors tied up with modern life: antibiotic use, exposure to chemicals, a diet high in sugars and processed foods, Caesarean section, formula feeding and time spent indoors.[6] Probiotic treatment for food allergies has shown promising results in babies and children.[7]

A real food, nutrient-dense diet may provide additional protection against food allergies and intolerances. If you suspect you have a food allergy, the first thing to do is remove processed food from your diet. Replace it with real food – meat, eggs, vegetables, fruit, nuts and olive oil. In my experience, most food allergies will disappear on this regime.

For dairy allergies, see page 101.

POINTS TO REMEMBER
- Gluten sensitivity can cause gut-related symptoms but may affect any tissue in the body.
- A trial of avoiding all grains is the first step to determine if you have gluten sensitivity.
- FODMAPs are another important group of substances that can cause food sensitivity; these respond well to dietary restriction.

Vegetarian and Vegan Diets

Vegetarian and vegan diets can be healthy but no healthier than a real-food low-carb diet.

Vegetarian diets seem to be increasing in popularity, and there's no doubt that a balanced vegetarian or vegan diet can provide many health benefits.

A vegetarian diet is of course based around plant foods. There are different types of vegetarian diet including:

- vegan: where only plant foods are eaten
- lacto: where dairy foods are included
- ovo-lacto: where dairy foods and eggs are included.

From my understanding, people decide to become vegetarian for one of three reasons:

1. ethical: concern about cruelty to animals
2. environmental: concern that animal farming is bad for the environment
3. health: belief that a vegetarian or vegan diet is better for their own health.

While the first and second reasons are too big to touch on here – and are not my primary domain – the third argument, that vegetarian and vegan diets are healthier than diets including meat, is not correct. That's not to say that a well-balanced vegan diet can't be healthy, but simply that good-quality meat, fish, eggs and dairy are superior sources of protein while also providing healthy fats along with other vitamins and minerals.

Whether or not a diet is healthy depends not so much on whether or not it includes meat, but rather how much unhealthy food it contains, such as sugars, processed foods and vegetable oils. A meat eater who eats mainly grain-fed processed meats along with large amounts of sugar and processed foods is likely to be considerably less healthy than a vegan who gets their nutrition from healthy plant sources.

Protein and vegetarians

Protein is one area where there is much debate between vegans and omnivores. As we've seen, when eaten, protein is broken down into amino acids. Proteins and amino acids are used for almost every metabolic process in the body. However, different proteins can vary greatly in the types of amino acids they contain.

In total, there are around 20 amino acids the human body uses to build proteins. These amino acids are classified as either non-essential, meaning we can make them ourselves, or essential, meaning we need to obtain them through our food. For optimal health, we need all the essential amino acids in the right ratios.

Animal protein sources, such as meat, fish, poultry, eggs and dairy, are similar to the protein found in our bodies and tend to contain a good balance of all the amino acids we need. These are considered complete sources of protein. On the other hand, plant protein sources, such as beans, lentils and nuts, are considered to be incomplete, as they lack one or more of the essential amino acids that your body needs. This means that different plant protein foods need to be combined in the same meal to 'complete' the protein and cover our amino acid needs.

Plants can provide most of the essential nutrients required for humans to function and in fact provide some important nutrients not found in animal foods, such as vitamin C, but there are a few nutrients that are only found in animals. These include vitamin B12, vitamin D, the omega-3 fatty acid DHA, haem iron and zinc.

Vegan diets

Vegan diets can include:

- fruit and vegetables
- breads, cereals and grains
- legumes (lentils, chickpeas and dried beans)
- soy foods (tofu and tempeh)
- nuts and seeds.

But vegan diets don't include:

- meat, poultry, fish and seafood
- dairy products
- eggs.

If you decide you want to go vegan, let's look at how you can ensure a healthy diet. A vegan diet requires careful planning to ensure all the necessary nutrients are present. There are certain areas where that can be a challenge, but provided these challenges are overcome, a vegan diet can be healthy.

Protein in vegan diets

As we've seen, the average adult probably requires at least 0.8–1.2 grams of protein per kilogram of body weight each day (and more if you're trying to bulk up, are pregnant or are aged over 60). Most people eating animal-based foods have no problem reaching those levels.

Those eating a vegan diet, however, have to make a conscious effort to obtain adequate protein. Beans, lentils, nuts and seeds, nut butters, tofu and tempeh can all up your daily protein intake. Vegetables such as kale, brussels sprouts, spinach and mushrooms can also be good sources of protein. Vegans should try to incorporate at least one or two of these foods into each meal to ensure adequate protein intake and 'completing' the protein.

Iron in vegan diets

There are many plant sources of iron, including legumes, tofu, nuts and seeds, whole grains (especially amaranth and quinoa), dried fruits and dark green leafy vegetables. However, the form of iron in plants (non-haem iron) isn't absorbed as well as the haem iron found in animal foods. This leaves vegans at risk of iron deficiency.

Vegans can lessen the risk of iron deficiency by including a food that's rich in vitamin C (e.g. berries, citrus fruit, kiwifruit, capsicum, tomato or broccoli) with meals to boost the absorption of iron from plant foods. Conversely, vegans should drink tea between meals rather than at the same time as their sources of iron, as it can interfere with iron absorption.

Vitamin B12 in vegan diets

Vitamin B12 (or cobalamin) is only found naturally in animal products. It plays a key role in the formation of DNA, as well as in normal brain and nervous system function through the synthesis of myelin. B12 deficiency can cause a range of symptoms, such as fatigue, lethargy, depression, poor memory, breathlessness, headaches and pale skin, especially in the elderly.

Some foods are fortified with vitamin B12, but vegans are generally advised to take a B12 supplement. Contrary to popular belief, mushrooms can't provide the B12 we need.

The fat-soluble vitamins (A, D and K2) and vegans

Vegan diets increase the risk of deficiencies in certain fat-soluble vitamins. Low-fat vegan diets further increase risk of these deficiencies, because sufficient fat must be eaten with every meal to absorb these vitamins from food.

Plant foods contain no vitamin A, but contain carotenoids, which we can convert into retinol, the form of vitamin A our bodies can use. Getting enough carotenoids is 12 to 24 times more difficult than obtaining retinol from animal foods. Many processed foods are fortified with vitamin A, however, so deficiency is uncommon.

The form of vitamin D our bodies need is D3 (cholecalciferol). We can make D3 from sunshine or obtain it from animal foods. The form of vitamin D found in plant foods is D2 (ergocalciferol). Our bodies can convert some D2 to D3, but D2 is less potent, doesn't last as long in the bloodstream, and may be harder to store in our body fat for rainy days and dark winters. If we spend enough time in the sun, we don't need to obtain any vitamin D from our diet at all (see pages 240–44), yet many people (regardless of chosen diet) are deficient. Most studies have found that vegans have lower blood levels of vitamin D3 and are more likely to drop to deficient levels during the winter months than meat-eaters.[1]

Vitamin K2 comes in many forms, but the essential form we need is called MK-4, which only exists in animal foods. The body can convert a little vitamin K1, which is abundant in many plant foods, into MK-4, but not nearly enough to fully meet our needs. Savvy vegans turn to natto (fermented soy), which contains a bacterial form of vitamin K our bodies can turn into MK-4 a little more easily.

Calcium in vegan diets

As a vegan diet doesn't include dairy products or fish, it's important for vegans to eat other calcium-rich foods. Some good plant sources of calcium are hard tofu, almonds, unhulled tahini (sesame seed paste) and green leafy vegetables such as kale and Asian greens (e.g. bok choy, Chinese broccoli).

Omega-3 fats in vegan diets

We've seen the importance of the omega-3 fats and of ensuring that the ratio of omega-6 to omega-3 stays within reasonable limits. Plants don't contain either of the two important omega-3 fats, EPA and DHA. Levels of EPA and DHA can be about 30 per cent lower in vegetarians and more than 50 per cent lower in vegans than in meat eaters.[2] This is primarily because the form of omega-3 (ALA) found in plant foods (flaxseed, chia seeds, walnut and soy) is very difficult for the body to convert into the DHA our brains need. Vegans should consider taking an algae-based omega-3 supplement.

POINTS TO REMEMBER

- Vegetarian diets, especially the vegan type, appear to be gaining in popularity.
- It's possible to eat a healthy vegan diet, but some supplementation will probably be necessary.

The Ketogenic Diet

How very low-carbohydrate diets work.

The ketogenic diet (KD) is a form of low-carb diet that reduces daily carb intake to around 20–30 grams a day, although there is considerable variation in the amount of carb restriction required. Such a low carb intake forces the body to rely on fat as the primary fuel source – a state known as nutritional ketosis. The fuel source produced by the breakdown of fat is called ketone bodies or simply ketones.

Clearly, a KD is quite strict and requires a big commitment to adhere to it for any significant period of time. Nevertheless, there are huge benefits to be gained.[1]

Who should consider a ketogenic diet?

If I or those around me had any of the following I would consider a ketogenic diet (KD) straight away, in combination with other treatments:

- morbid obesity
- type 2 diabetes
- metabolic syndrome
- an autoimmune disease, e.g. rheumatoid arthritis, inflammatory bowel disease
- intractable epilepsy
- a neurodegenerative disease, e.g. dementia, Alzheimer's, Parkinson's disease
- traumatic brain injury (TBI)
- multiple sclerosis (MS)
- cancer
- chronic fatigue syndrome
- fibromyalgia
- ADHD
- autism
- PCOS/infertility.

I would regard all of the above conditions serious enough to warrant drastic action. I would try a KD for two to three months – I think that's long enough to see if there is any benefit. If there was a positive response, then I might well choose to continue with the diet and make it a permanent part of my lifestyle. An alternative approach would be to start with a KD to get the maximum positive effect, then slowly add measured amounts of carbohydrate each week to see what level of carb intake the body can tolerate while still maintaining the benefits.

What food is allowed in a ketogenic diet?

The carb restriction is so severe that the only carbs will come from green vegetables and a few nuts. Otherwise, it entails eating real foods such as grass-fed meat, oily fish, eggs, butter, liver and other organ meats, and coconut and olive oils, and drinking bone broths, water, tea (green or herbal), or coffee with cream or coconut milk/cream.

How to know if you're in nutritional ketosis

The aim of the ketogenic diet is to reach a state of nutritional ketosis where ketones are the primary fuel source. There's no guaranteed level of carb intake that will ensure ketosis – we're all different. Many people can tell when they are in ketosis by their breath, which has a distinctive sweet smell of ketones.

If you want greater precision, it's possible to measure the ketones in your urine with colour-changing indicator papers, a finger-prick test with a blood ketone meter, or a small device you blow into to measure ketones in the breath.

Is a ketogenic diet safe? What about ketoacidosis?

The KD produces blood ketone levels up to 3 or 4 mmol/L, which are safe levels. Some people confuse nutritional ketosis with ketoacidosis. The latter is a serious medical emergency seen only in type 1 diabetics, and is associated with blood ketone levels three to five times higher than those seen in nutritional ketosis – so it is not a concern for those on a ketogenic diet.

KETO 'FLU'

When you first commence a KD, it's not unusual to feel awful for a few days. This is known as keto 'flu' and usually lasts a week or two at the most. You feel fatigued and may have some sugar cravings, muscle aches, brain fog and/or difficulty getting to sleep. Don't worry about it, but rather see as it as a positive – an indication that your system is changing. One possible contributing factor is low sodium so make sure you get plenty of salt.

Once you're past that adaptation stage and fully fuelled by fats, you'll most likely have reduced appetite and increased energy.

Muscle cramps

The only other common side effect of a KD is nocturnal muscle cramps, mainly affecting the large leg muscles. The exact cause of these cramps is debated, but could be due to low salt intake. A KD with zero processed foods is low in salt, so you may need to increase your salt intake by adding salt to your foods. The other possible culprit is magnesium, so you might want to try a magnesium supplement to combat the cramps if the increased salt doesn't do the trick.

POINTS TO REMEMBER
- A ketogenic diet is a safe, extremely low-carb diet.
- Those with serious medical conditions should consider it and discuss with their doctor.
- Ketone levels can be measured.

Fasting

Fasting can be easy and offers real health benefits.

If you'd told me a couple of years ago that fasting might be a healthy option, I would have laughed in your face. How could anyone think that depriving yourself of nutrients for an extended period could be beneficial for your health? Anyway, I would have said, no one in their right mind could do it because you'd get too hungry. As I learn more and more about the workings of the human body, though, I'm increasingly convinced that fasting, whether intermittent or regular, can be great for your health. When you think about it, humans have been 'fasting' for centuries, whether as part of their hunter-gatherer lifestyle or for spiritual reasons.

One of the leading advocates of fasting, Dr Jason Fung, author of *The Obesity Code* and (with Jimmy Moore) *The Complete Guide to Fasting*, explains it very simply. As we've seen, calorie-restriction diets fail because the body adapts to the lower intake. We know that insulin leads to fat storage: if we produce insulin, fat will be stored. If we deprive the body of insulin, fat will be mobilised from our fat stores.

One way of reducing the insulin in our body is to reduce our intake of carbs, especially from added sugar and processed foods. This is effective for most people, and leads to increased weight loss and normalisation of other metabolic measures such as blood glucose, triglycerides, HDL cholesterol and liver function.

An even more effective way of reducing insulin is by fasting. When we fast, we stop producing insulin. As a result, our energy stores are mobilised, initially from the glycogen (glucose) stores in the liver and then, after a period of time, from our fat stores. No food, no insulin, so it makes sense that fasting will result in weight loss.

Dr Fung lists seven advantages of fasting:

1. simplicity
2. affordability

3. convenience
4. its cheat days
5. powerful effects
6. flexibility
7. versatility – it can be added to any diet.

Which leaves two remaining questions: is it healthy and can anyone do it? The answer to the first question would appear to be yes, at least for fasts of no longer than few days with a decent period in between. Pregnant and breastfeeding women shouldn't fast, and it's not advised for children and the elderly.

How long to fast

Fasting can be anything from a few hours to a few days. We all fast overnight and break our fast with our 'break-fast'. That might be a daily 12-hour fast. Some will increase that by having an early dinner and late breakfast, stretching it out to maybe 14–16 hours. Alternatively, you could skip breakfast altogether, which would give you maybe an 18-hour fast. A popular regime is daily fasting for 18 hours this way, and fitting in all your food intake into a 6-hour window, for example 1 p.m. till 7 p.m. This is known as time-restricted eating or TRE.

Another option is the alternate-day fast or the popular 5:2 fast, where you eat minimal calories two days a week while eating a normal healthy real food diet the other five days. Then there is the option of the longer fast – 24 hours or two-, three- or four-day fasts. Impossible, you say. Surprisingly not. Yes, you get occasional hunger pangs, but they pass and can be quelled with some water, black coffee, green tea or bone broth, all of which are allowed in a fast.

A lot of people will tell you how great they feel during a fast – I know it's hard to imagine if you haven't done it. Give it a try and see how you go, but check with your GP first to ensure it's safe for you to try a longer fast.

How I use fasts

I do regular 12-, 14- or 16-hour fasts, which I don't find difficult on a low-sugar, real-food diet because I'm rarely hungry. I try to eat only when I'm hungry rather than at a specific time. That's certainly a challenge socially, as a lot of socialising revolves around meals – and we're all social animals. So I try to adjust my eating depending on my social commitments. If I have a breakfast meeting, I might skip dinner the night before or lunch that day. Likewise, if I have a lunch engagement, I'll always skip breakfast. I occasionally do longer 24- or 36-hour fasts with just fluids, and have had no problems with them.

POINTS TO REMEMBER
- Fasting is an interesting option for those who wish to improve their health.
- Fasting can be regular, with a prolonged period without food each day, or intermittent, involving one- to four-day fasts.
- Intermittent fasting appears to be both safe and healthy, but check with your GP before you begin.

Female-specific Issues

*Women can find relief from specific health issues
with a real-food, low-carb diet.*

There are a number of specific issues related to women's health and diet
and lifestyle. These include PCOS, gestational diabetes, osteoporosis and
iron deficiency.

Fertility

Fertility issues in women aren't generally regarded as diet-related, but I have
no doubt that diet plays a role. A poor diet high in inflammatory foods such
as sugar, processed foods and vegetable oils can create a state of chronic
inflammation that can interfere with fertility. Fertility experts are slowly coming to the same conclusion, and some are now incorporating dietary advice
to reduce carbohydrate intake as a part of their management program.[1]

Recent research from the Delaware Institute for Reproductive Medicine
found that women with lower carbohydrate intake had four times the
pregnancy success rates of those on standard diets. The US trial involved
120 women undergoing IVF. Researchers split the women into two groups,
depending on the balance of protein and carbohydrate in their diet. In
total, 58 per cent of those in the 'low-carb' group went on to have a baby.
In the 'high-carb' group, just 11 per cent achieved success.[2]

The most common cause of female infertility is polycystic ovary syndrome (PCOS).

Polycystic ovary syndrome (PCOS)

PCOS is one of the most common endocrine (hormone system) disorders
among women of reproductive age. In PCOS, a hormonal balance affects
ovulation. Instead of an egg being released from one of the ovary follicles
each month, the egg fails to mature and the follicle instead forms a small
cyst. This process occurs repeatedly, until the ovaries eventually contain
dozens of cysts.

The symptoms vary from person to person, and some women are virtually symptomless, but the hallmarks of PCOS are insulin resistance and high blood insulin levels (hyperinsulinemia). Other common symptoms include:

- obesity
- menstrual irregularities such as amenorrhoea (skipped periods) and menorrhagia (heavy periods) as a result of not ovulating
- masculine features, such as excessive facial and body hair, acne, male-pattern baldness, and deep voice, due to increased ovarian production of testosterone and 'male' hormones
- acanthosis nigricans (skin tags and darkened pigment in skin folds, such as the armpits, groin, thighs and neck), a sign of insulin resistance and hyperinsulinemia
- depression.

Young women are three to five times more likely to develop diabetes if they suffer from PCOS.[3]

Medical management of PCOS has traditionally consisted of insulin-sensitising medications such as metformin, along with stress management, exercise, support groups and supplements.

As insulin resistance and hyperinsulinemia are the underlying factors leading to PCOS, it seems logical that a low-carb diet (<50 grams of carbohydrate per day) should be the front-line treatment of PCOS. Limiting refined carbohydrates, sugars and processed oils can result in lower insulin levels, increase insulin sensitivity, and balance the endocrine system, allowing ovulation and a normal menstrual cycle.

Many women have been able to manage or reverse their PCOS symptoms, including infertility, through a low-carb diet.

Pregnancy

Diet and exercise are both important factors in pregnancy.

Diet during pregnancy

What a pregnant woman eats affects the nutrition and development of her baby. Diets high in sugar increase the likelihood of the mother developing gestational diabetes (see page 188) and also affect the blood sugar levels of the baby. This means the baby will expect sugar from the moment he or she pops out into the real world, so the poor kid is already in trouble from day one.

The same basic principles of good nutrition apply for pregnant women – lots of real food including meat, fish, eggs, vegetables, nuts and olive oil, with a minimum of sugar, processed foods and vegetable oils. Food tastes often change during pregnancy and cravings for sugary foods are not uncommon. It's important to try to resist sugar cravings, though, because eating sugar will only make you want to eat more of it. Maintaining stable blood glucose levels is vital for both mother and baby.

No one's suggesting that a pregnant mother should go on a severe low-carb diet such as a ketogenic diet – we just don't have enough evidence one way or the other about these diets during pregnancy. I'm not saying no carbs, just keep it lowish, focus on healthy carbs in fruits and vegetables, and avoid the empty calories in soft drinks, confectionery and junk food.

In recent years, doctors have expressed some concern about certain foods during pregnancy, especially those associated with listeria infections, which can be damaging to the foetus. As a consequence, many pregnant women avoid foods such as raw fish and meat, raw sprouts, soft mould-ripened cheeses and processed meats. I would certainly not recommend avoiding all meat and fish as there are numerous health benefits from eating both. It's important to ensure good hygiene and high-quality produce.

Alcohol and caffeine are big no-nos during pregnancy. Small amounts of both (one drink a day) would seem to be okay, but a complete alcohol ban during pregnancy seems to me to be a good idea.

Exercise during pregnancy
Exercise is extremely beneficial during pregnancy. While pregnancy is probably not the best time to commence an intense exercise routine, most women who had been exercising at a high level before pregnancy can continue to exercise for at least part of the pregnancy. As I write this, there is much publicity about tennis player Mandy Minella playing at Wimbledon while four and a half months pregnant! Care should be taken to avoid overheating, so avoiding exercise during the heat of the day is probably a good idea.

For those not already exercising at a high level before pregnancy, regular mild to moderate exercise, such as walking or swimming, is very beneficial.

Gestational diabetes

Gestational diabetes (GD) is a type of diabetes triggered by pregnancy. Women with GD didn't have diabetes before they were pregnant and it generally goes away after the birth, at least temporarily.

Like all other kinds of diabetes, though, GD has been getting more and more common. GD is more common in older mothers, women with a family history of type 2 diabetes, and women who were overweight before their pregnancy. A woman who has GD during one pregnancy is likely to have it in later pregnancies. Once a woman has had GD, she's at a much higher risk of developing type 2 diabetes in the future – and so are her kids.

Most women who have GD deliver healthy babies, but untreated or uncontrolled blood sugar levels can cause problems for both mother and baby. Babies whose mothers have GD tend to be large (and may need to be delivered by caesarean).

The first indication of GD may be the presence of sugar in a regular urine test, but is more likely an abnormal result in the glucose tolerance test (GTT) performed routinely about halfway through pregnancy.

What causes gestational diabetes?

GD occurs in women who already have a degree of insulin resistance – usually unrecognised – before the pregnancy. Insulin resistance increases during pregnancy, which on top of the pre-pregnancy insulin resistance can be enough to cause GD.

Prevention and treatment of gestational diabetes

Given that women who develop GD had some degree of insulin resistance beforehand, it's important to recognise and correct that insulin resistance as early as possible. Occasionally there are indicators of possible insulin resistance, such as abdominal obesity (an apple shape) and abnormal blood tests (elevated fasting insulin, high triglycerides or low HDL), but there are often no obvious signs in the early stages of insulin resistance.

Whether the insulin resistance is recognised before the pregnancy or only after GD is diagnosed, the two key components of management are diet and exercise. Regular exercise has been shown to modify insulin resistance, so regular mild to moderate exercise is recommended.[4] Sugar intake should be reduced, with a focus on real foods and reduction in processed foods, especially refined carbohydrates, and vegetable oils.

Osteoporosis

Osteoporosis is a common disease affecting more than 1 million Australians. Although the majority are women, it's important to note that men can also develop osteoporosis, especially in older age. This disease makes bones brittle, leading to a higher risk of fractures. These fractures significantly increase the risk of death for older adults, sometimes by a factor of two or three.

Osteoporosis occurs when bones lose minerals such as calcium faster than the body can replace them, causing a loss of bone density. Osteopenia is a precursor to osteoporosis, and both are diagnosed through bone mineral density scans with a DEXA machine (see Toolkit 2). It can be totally asymptomatic until a fracture occurs.

Women are at a greater risk of developing osteoporosis because oestrogen levels drop rapidly during menopause. When oestrogen levels fall, the bones lose calcium and other minerals much faster, and bone is lost at a rate of about 2 per cent per year for several years after menopause.

Risk factors for developing osteoporosis include a family history, low calcium intake, low vitamin D levels, certain chronic diseases (thyroid problems, malabsorption conditions such as coeliac disease, rheumatoid arthritis), certain medications (corticosteroids), early menopause, and lifestyle factors such as lack of exercise, smoking, excess alcohol intake and obesity.

Adults should have a calcium intake of 1000 mg per day, and this should increase to 1300 mg per day for women over 50 and men over 70. This calcium should ideally come from food – calcium supplements have not been found to be helpful in preventing osteoporosis. Dairy is well known as a good source of calcium, but there are plenty of other sources for those who can't tolerate dairy, including fish with bones (tinned salmon and sardines), nuts (almonds, hazelnuts, pistachios), vegetables (broccoli, kale), figs, beans, seaweeds, sesame seeds, tofu and bone broth.

A low vitamin D level is an important risk factor for developing osteoporosis, and is best managed through increased exposure to the sun (see page 236).

Inflammation has also been added to the list of possible causes of osteoporosis. Research has shown that inflammatory markers in the blood are related to bone loss and broken bones in both women and men.[5] A recent study indicated a high-inflammatory diet had a greater negative impact on the younger women in the study. Caucasian women younger than 63 who ate a high-inflammatory diet were 50 per cent more likely to fracture a hip than those on a low-inflammatory diet.[6] Women in this study eating a low-inflammatory diet also lost bone slower than women on a high-inflammatory diet.

A diet of real foods with low sugar and minimal processed foods, especially no vegetable oils, is recommended. Weightbearing exercise is the other important contributor to reducing the risk of osteoporosis (see page 216).

Iron deficiency

Iron deficiency or at least iron depletion is extremely common in women of all ages, but more so in menstruating women. Iron deficiency anaemia is defined in women as a haemoglobin level of less than 120 grams per litre. Iron depletion is indicated by a normal haemoglobin level (>120 g/L) but serum ferritin level (an indicator of iron stores) of less than 30 µg/ml.

Someone with iron-deficiency anaemia typically experiences fatigue, weakness, shortness of breath, reduced exercise tolerance and pallor.

There are three possible causes of iron deficiency:

1. insufficient dietary intake
2. inadequate iron absorption
3. increased iron loss, i.e. through bleeding or menstruation.

Examples of iron-rich foods include meat, eggs, leafy green vegetables and iron-fortified foods, but it's important to note that absorption is much greater from meat (which provides haem iron) than vegetables (non-haem iron). This puts vegetarians and vegans at greater risk of iron deficiency. Absorption can be improved by eating the iron source with vitamin C, and inhibited by drinking tea.

If you're diagnosed as iron-deficient or iron-depleted, your GP should first ensure that there's no source of unexplained bleeding. If that's ruled out, the best approach is to try to increase your intake of dietary iron (especially from red meat and liver), preferably eaten with a source of vitamin C (such as red capsicum), and avoiding tannin-rich drinks such as tea.

Iron supplements can be helpful. The best are ferrous sulfate or ferrous succinate, but many people don't tolerate iron supplements well.

POINTS TO REMEMBER
- PCOS is a disease of insulin resistance and should be managed with a low-carb diet.
- Good nutrition is extremely important during pregnancy. Gestational diabetes needs careful management with a low-carb diet.
- Exercise and diet are the keys to managing osteoporosis.
- Regular intake of iron-rich foods is important to prevent iron-deficiency anaemia.

Feeding Kids

Kids need to eat real food to ensure good health well into adulthood.

At least a quarter of Australian kids are overweight or obese. In fact, it's probably more. In certain areas of the country, more than 50 per cent of primary school children are overweight. The numbers appear to be increasing, and the projected figures for 2025 look pretty depressing.

Overweight and obese children in Australia

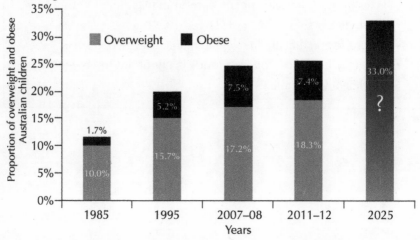

Source: Leung, J., Funder, J., *Obesity Australia*, 2014[1]

We know that fat kids tend to become fat adults – once you're overweight it's very hard to get the weight off. The best solution is not to let your kids get overweight. Simple, eh!

We also know that insulin resistance, which is the key factor in the development of chronic diseases such as type 2 diabetes, develops as a result of long-term exposure to large amounts of carbohydrates in the diet. So the best solution is not to expose them to those high levels of carbohydrates from birth.

What should kids eat?

As parents, we have a huge responsibility for the health and wellbeing of our children. I have to admit that I didn't do a great job with my own kids' nutrition. They had too many empty calories – fruit juice, sports drinks, chocolate milk, puréed fruit, flavoured yoghurts, muesli bars and so on. 'Treats' involved a visit to Maccas or some ice cream.

Aaaargh! If only I could have my time again, knowing what I know now. Don't make the same mistake. Hopefully, I'll do a better job as a grandparent!

My kids seem to have survived their second-rate nutrition, although one of our boys had significant issues with obesity until at about the age of eleven he decided for himself that he would eat no more junk food. He lost about 10 kilograms and was able to excel at the sports he'd always loved but had never been able to play well before. His academic performance improved as well.

The same principles apply to both children and their parents and can be summed up by one simple phrase:

> Eat real food

Give your kids plenty of meat, fish, dairy, fruit and vegetables, nuts and olive oil, and as little as possible of sugar and related foods, processed carbohydrates and vegetable oils.

Even the average Australian two- to three-year-old child is having about 32 grams (8 teaspoons) of added sugar a day, in addition to the natural sugar in fruit and dairy. That amount more than doubles by the time they're teenagers, and large numbers of teenagers are having more than 120 grams (30 teaspoons) a day.

Avoiding sugar is a pretty good start, but as any parent knows, it's easier said than done. That's why it is important to start early.

Breastfeeding

Breastmilk is the ideal nutrition for a newborn baby, so every attempt should be made to breastfeed.

Some mothers find it easy – the baby latches on straight away and everything goes smoothly. I have to say that in my experience that's the exception rather than the rule. Too little milk (or too much), cracked nipples, mastitis, blocked milk ducts and engorged breasts can all make initiating breastfeeding a difficult, painful, stressful experience. Add to that a new mother's natural anxiety and lack of sleep, and it's a wonder that so many mothers actually succeed with breastfeeding.

Despite all of these possible initial difficulties, I would strongly urge mothers to persevere. Breastfeeding is best for your baby and feeding creates a wonderful bond between mother and baby. As a father, I was always a little bit jealous of my wife having that relationship!

Fortunately, these days there is usually plenty of professional support to help you with breastfeeding. Nursing staff both at the hospital and at the local child and maternity centre have enormous experience, and there are even lactation specialists to help. Be patient, it can take days or even weeks to get things going smoothly.

While you're breastfeeding, it's really important to meet your own nutritional needs. This can be challenging, as you're likely to be time-poor and constantly exhausted. The last thing you'll feel like doing is spending significant amounts of time preparing and cooking food, so the temptation may be to live off fast food during that period. Not all takeaway foods are necessarily of poor nutritional quality (see page 143) and Asian takeaways in particular can offer plenty of healthy options.

Another option is for you and/or your partner to cook up a bunch of healthy casseroles and other dishes while you're pregnant and freeze them for use during these difficult first few months. Of course, any fresh meals provided by helpful grandparents, neighbours and friends will be very gratefully received!

If, despite your best efforts, you are unable to breastfeed or have to give up after a while, don't stress. Your baby can still thrive. Commercial infant formulas are the best alternative to breastfeeding, and are designed to be similar in content to breastmilk. Unfortunately, they contain a few too many vegetable oils for my liking, but they are all the same in that regard.

The majority of infant formulas are cow's milk-based and contain the milk sugar lactose. These formulas are usually then fortified with extra vitamins, minerals, fats and protein to mimic the content of breastmilk. Some babies don't tolerate these cow's-milk formulas, not because they're lactose intolerant (babies aren't lactose intolerant at birth), but because they're allergic to one of the milk proteins. In that case, a hydrolysed protein or goat's milk formula are probably preferable to a soy one.

If you're having trouble choosing the right formula, I suggest asking your infant welfare nurse or another expert for advice.

Introducing solids

When to introduce solids on top of breastmilk (or formula) is a controversial question. There's no set rule, but usually at five or six months the baby will be looking for something extra. They won't find the milk feeds satisfying, or might no longer sleep through the night.

Around that time, get out the steamer and the blender and start preparing some real food for your baby. Start with a teaspoon of puréed food and slowly increase their intake over the following days. Food texture is really important, so start off with it as smooth as possible then gradually introduce lumps.

The best food to start with is vegetables, so maybe some puréed pumpkin or carrots initially, and then a wider range of vegetables (broccoli, beans, zucchini, etc.). Once the baby is tolerating puréed vegetables, it's time to add eggs (scrambled is perfect) and meat to the purée. Fruit can then be added, but keep to small amounts. Try to avoid processed baby foods and fruit juices, which are all high in sugar.

An alternative approach now gaining popularity is baby-led weaning. Here, instead of blending special foods, babies are allowed to self-feed from family foods in their whole form. The emphasis is on allowing kids to choose what, and how much, they eat and for them to be part of family mealtimes. At around six months, the majority of babies develop the motor skills required for self-feeding, including being able to sit up unsupported, bring food to their mouths, and chew and swallow food.

Supporters of this approach suggest that it offers several benefits for babies, including better appetite control, a more varied diet and even motor skill development. Initial research suggests that baby-led weaning may foster positive eating behaviour and potentially desirable weight gain, but further research is required.

Toddlers and older kids

By now I am sure you are getting the picture – real foods, not processed stuff.

When kids live off a diet of sugary drinks and snacks, and processed foods, they become accustomed to sweetness. It becomes the norm. This, of course, is what the food industry wants. Manufacturers make sure that all processed foods are sweet (just look at tomato and barbecue sauces, for example), so kids aren't happy unless their food is sweet. The more processed sweetened food they eat, the more they crave it.

As we know, after a meal full of sugar and starches, blood sugar levels spike, followed soon after by a large plunge leading to low blood sugar levels, which in turn leads to hunger and the desire for more food. Avoiding sugar and starches, and eating the proteins and healthy fats in real food, results in stable blood glucose levels and a marked reduction in hunger.

The junk food industry spends millions of dollars each year marketing its products to children, so it can be difficult to convince kids that real food is the way to go. There's lots of peer pressure from their friends, too, who might be heading off regularly to a fast-food outlet, or drinking soft drinks or sports drinks. Kids hate to be different and don't want to draw attention to themselves by 'eating funny'.

There are plenty of challenges. It's hard enough getting adults to eat vegetables, let alone kids, so we need to make the vegetables fun with innovative presentation. Use different colours, textures, shapes and sizes to make food interesting. Make faces out of food, or let the kids do it.

Here are some other general ideas that could make feeding kids easier:

- Eat as a family.
- Avoid distractions such as TV and devices while eating.
- Don't rush eating. Family meals are a great time for conversation and laughs.
- Don't bribe your kids to eat.
- Introduce new foods small amounts at a time. Be patient. They might not like it first time, but don't push it. Just try again later.
- Disguise disliked foods (e.g. liver) among others.
- Use alternatives such as homemade tomato sauce instead of bought sauce.
- Use butter and salt for flavour.
- Allow occasional blowouts such as children's parties.

School lunches

School lunches can be very challenging. Traditionally, we send our kids off with a sandwich, a drink (usually fruit juice) and a biscuit or muesli bar. Lunches were my task at home and that was pretty much what I was giving my kids back in the day.

Healthy school lunches aren't difficult to prepare, but they do need a little imagination. Use lunchboxes with little compartments and fill them with real food: cheese cubes, cherry tomatoes, ham, carrots, hard-boiled eggs. Use cold meat, such as roast beef, as a 'wrap' and put cheese and vegetables inside.

I don't have the space here to give you lots of suggestions regarding kids' lunches and kids' food in general, but there are lots of good websites with great information. I really like the Ditch the Carbs website, www.ditchthe-carbs.com. Its fabulous creator Libby provides a wealth of information not just on kids' lunches but a whole range of low-carb topics. Libby has been kind enough to let me use one of her infographics and there are lots more.

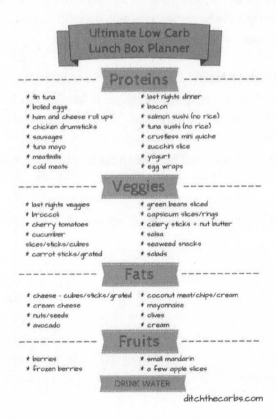

Ultimate Low Carb Lunch Box Planner

Proteins
* tin tuna
* boiled eggs
* ham and cheese roll ups
* chicken drumsticks
* sausages
* tuna mayo
* meatballs
* cold meats
* last nights dinner
* bacon
* salmon sushi (no rice)
* tuna sushi (no rice)
* crustless mini quiche
* zucchini slice
* yogurt
* egg wraps

Veggies
* last nights veggies
* broccoli
* cherry tomatoes
* cucumber slices/sticks/cubes
* carrot sticks/grated
* green beans sliced
* capsicum slices/rings
* celery sticks + nut butter
* salsa
* seaweed snacks
* salads

Fats
* cheese - cubes/sticks/grated
* cream cheese
* nuts/seeds
* avocado
* coconut meat/chips/cream
* mayonnaise
* olives
* cream

Fruits
* berries
* frozen berries
* small mandarin
* a few apple slices

DRINK WATER

ditchthecarbs.com

What should kids drink?

Sugar-sweetened beverages such as soft drinks and sports drinks make up a significant proportion of the ridiculously high amount of added sugar consumed by teenagers in this country. I believe that these drinks are a major contributing factor to our epidemics of obesity and type 2 diabetes.

The best way of stopping kids drinking this rubbish is never letting them start. I would prefer it if your kids never had a soft drink or sports drink, although I suppose the odd can of Coke or bottle of Gatorade won't do too much harm.

The best drinks for kids are water and milk. If they find water too bland, try adding some berries or lemon or lime into it – maybe with some mint. Plain full fat milk is best. Avoid flavoured milks and please, please don't give your kids low-fat milk – studies have shown links to more obesity with skim milk than the full-fat variety.[2] There was never any science behind the low-fat milk recommendations anyway.

And what about diet drinks such as Diet Coke or Diet Pepsi? While they may be marginally better than the full-strength drinks, they have their own problems (see page 165).

More information

For a full list of resources see my website, fatlotofgood.com.au. The best book for kids' nutrition is *Super Food for Superchildren* by Professor Tim Noakes and his South African colleagues. I've had the privilege of being a long-time friend of Tim's, and he's been a pioneer in advocating his Banting (low-carb) diet in his home country. His first book, *Real Meal Revolution*, was on the bestseller list for months in South Africa, and this follow-up book of information and recipes especially for kids is outstanding.

POINTS TO REMEMBER
- More than a quarter of Australian kids are overweight or obese, mainly thanks to a poor diet full of sugar and processed foods.
- Get your kids to eat real food.
- Getting your kids eating well is a challenge for the whole family.

Diet and Sports Performance

Carbs are supposedly 'king' – but is that still the case?

Back in the 1980s, I co-authored the first Australian sports nutrition book, *Food for Sport*, with dietitian Karen Inge. The main message of that book was that carbohydrates were the primary fuel for the athlete. And so it stayed for 30 years. Any serious (or recreational for that matter) athlete was eating a diet full of carbs, carb loading before running a marathon, and recovering with carbs. Carbs were in, fat was out. Sports drinks were in, water was out. Now, with the benefit of hindsight, we can see the adverse effects of high sugar and carb intake, such as insulin resistance, metabolic syndrome, type 2 diabetes and other chronic diseases.

We've usually associated poor nutrition with sedentary behaviour, but over the past 20–30 years we have had our finest athletes on a very 'unhealthy' diet. It will be interesting to follow this generation of carb-loaded athletes and observe the health consequences as they move through middle age. Multiple Tour de France winner Chris Froome was recently quoted on the consequences of consuming lots of carbohydrates on race days: 'It'll be three gels an hour towards the end. Plenty of riders get teeth problems from constant gels and drinks. I've had my fair share of fillings.'[1]

In the last few years, more and more athletes have been incorporating fats as their primary or secondary fuel. Diets like the LCHF, paleo and ketogenic diets have become popular especially among endurance and ultra-endurance athletes. Many athletes have claimed in media stories to have improved their endurance and ultra-endurance performance after switching to a diet primarily fuelled by fat, although scientific evidence is still largely lacking.

This has created huge controversy with the fat-as-fuel advocates lined up against the traditional carb-is-king supporters. As with everything in nutrition, they both have evidence to support their cases, and there's probably room for both regimes in sport.

The traditional high-carb athlete diet

Carbohydrate ingested in food and drink is stored as glycogen in the liver and primarily in the muscle. The muscle glycogen acts as a carbohydrate store and is available to fuel activity.

Even with a concerted attempt to maximise glycogen stores in the days leading up to competition (carb loading), there's a limit to the amount that can be stored. In addition, after exercising for a period of time (about two hours in most cases), the muscle glycogen stores become depleted and need to be restored. The challenge for the athlete is how to replenish the stores while exercising. The tendency is to use simple, easily digestible forms of carbohydrates such as sports drinks and gels.

There's no doubt that carbohydrate is the most effective fuel for high-intensity activity. Carbohydrate oxidation produces more energy per molecule than fat oxidation. My main concern with the emphasis on carbohydrates for fuel, however, is the health issues we've learnt are associated with high carb intake.

Fat as fuel for athletes

While fat can't provide as much energy as carbs, it has one big advantage – there are unlimited stores of fat in the body. Even the thinnest athlete has enough fat to use as fuel for many hours of activity.

When the body is deprived of carbohydrate for fuel, as with a low-carb or ketogenic diet (see page 179), it uses other fuel, mainly ketone bodies, aka ketones. After a period of time, usually one to two weeks (but sometimes longer), the body 'adapts' to this new fuel and starts to oxidise fat for fuel rather than carbs. During that period of adaptation, the athlete will often feel fatigued and unwell, and may struggle to perform at a high level, a phenomenon known as 'keto flu' (see page 181).

There are a number of advantages to using fat as a fuel, one of them being weight loss. It's always surprised me how many highly trained athletes are still a few kilograms overweight, despite their large exercise loads. I guess it's another example of 'You can't outrun a bad diet'. Invariably, when changing from a carb-dominant diet to a fat-dominant one, the athlete loses weight. Initially that's because of the water loss associated with reduced glycogen stores, but soon fat is lost. Reduced appetite associated with using fat as the major fuel source can also be a factor in weight loss.

The weight-loss aspect is particularly appealing to athletes, as the weight is not lost from muscle but from fat, thereby improving the power-to-weight ratio.

Weight loss is very important in those sports where there are weight limits, such as boxing, wrestling, martial arts, lightweight rowing and horseracing. Gymnasts and divers, for whom a low percentage of body fat is an advantage, also find the lower-carb, higher-fat diet helpful in weight control.

The other area where fat-adapted athletes really notice a change is in recovery after a hard workout. One of the major limiting factors to sporting performance is the inability to recover fully after training in time to do more training. Being fat-adapted leads to significantly less post-exercise muscle and joint soreness. This is thought to be due to the reduction in inflammation when sugars and processed foods are avoided and healthy fats eaten.

Carbs aren't required to increase muscle mass. The most important nutrient for someone wanting to bulk up is protein. For these people, the daily intake of protein, which must be of high quality, should be in the region of 1.5–2 grams per kilogram of body weight.

Should you eat carbs or fats?

The controversy over the best combination of fuels for athletic performance continues. Many sports nutrition experts are sticking to the carb-is-king philosophy and are very dismissive of those promoting fat as the preferred fuel. As with most controversies the truth lies somewhere in the middle.

The best fuel for you depends on a number of factors:

1. Your genetic make-up.
2. The duration of the exercise you do.
3. The intensity of your exercise.

It varies from individual to individual, but fat can fuel activity of about 70–80 per cent of your aerobic capacity (maximum oxygen output or VO2 max). At exercise intensities beyond that, carbs are required for maximum performance.

Generally speaking, the longer the duration and the lower the intensity of your exercise, the more likely it is that fat is your preferred fuel. For example, in ultra-distance running (such as 100-mile races), fat is the pre-ferred fuel, as you can maintain a moderate intensity of exercise for lengthy periods without having to constantly refuel as you would if you were rely-ing on carbs. In contrast, an activity such as running an 800-metre race requires carbs to fuel the high intensity.

WARNER'S LOW-CARB WIN

Back in 2013, Australian cricketer David Warner was overweight and not as fit as he should have been. It was another example of an athlete training and playing virtually 24/7 and yet still having a higher body fat content than he should. While we were touring in India, Davey decided to do something about it. He stopped drinking alcohol, severely reduced his carb intake and hit the gym.

Until then, his diet hadn't been terrible, but he was eating quite a lot of carbs in the belief that he could burn them off. With the reduction in carbs, he lost a significant amount of weight and soon went from being one of those in the team with the highest skinfold (body fat) measurements to one of the lowest.

Davey did love his carbs – so we agreed on Carb Sunday, one day a week when he could indulge in carbs. Davey would initially try to stretch it and tell me it was Sunday somewhere in the world. When he started telling me that on Tuesdays, I drew the line!

Intermittent high-intensity sports

Many sports, such as ball games (football, basketball, hockey, etc.) and road cycling, are a mixture of steady-state activity interspersed with bursts of high activity – a footballer sprinting for the ball, a road cyclist sprint-ing or climbing. The athlete using only fats as fuel will often complain that they lack the required energy to complete the high-intensity tasks, while the carb-fuelled athlete is constantly having to top up their fuel while also missing the benefits of the fat-fuelled athlete such as improved recovery.

The solution to this dilemma being adopted by elite athletes in various sports is to tailor their nutrition to their daily needs. An athlete having a steady lower-intensity training day, for example, would load up on healthy fats because high-intensity exercise isn't required. On days of competition or intense training, on the other hand, the athlete would supplement their fat intake with some readily available carbs, either the day before or the morning of the exercise, and then have carbs available during the game or training.

An AFL, rugby league or union or soccer player will have a basic low-carb, high-healthy-fat diet to maximise their ability to use fats as fuel, and then on both their one or two intense training days, as well as the day before and the morning of match day, will have a moderate amount of carbs in their meals.

The idea behind this is to get the best of both worlds: to have their fat-as-fuel system up and running, allowing them to use fat for their base needs; and then use the carbs to cover the high-intensity activity. This is known as the hybrid system of fuelling, or the 'train low, compete high' system. For those in need of this type of approach, there's a great deal of individual variation in preferred fuel usage, so it's a matter of trying different regimes to see which one suits them best.

I hope that the long-term effects of athletes reducing their traditional high-carb intake will be a reduction in the development of insulin resistance and its associated problems – obesity, type 2 diabetes, chronic disease.

POINTS TO REMEMBER
- Traditionally, athletes have used carbs as their major fuel source but recently there has been increased interest in the use of our unlimited fat stores as a fuel.
- Fat seems to be the preferred fuel for moderate-intensity endurance activity, while carbs are required for shorter-term high-intensity sports.
- The hybrid or 'train low, compete high' regime is becoming popular among elite athletes involved in sports with a mixture of endurance and high-intensity activities.

PART VI

The S-entials of Healthy Living

So far I've focused on what we should and shouldn't be eating. It's taken up the majority of this book because it's complex and often misunderstood. But there are other important components of a healthy lifestyle, what I call the 'S-entials' of healthy living:

- *Reduce SUGAR and processed foods.*
- *Avoid SEDENTARY behaviour.*
- *Achieve more good-quality SLEEP.*
- *Reduce STRESS.*
- *Get moderate SUN exposure.*
- *Don't SMOKE.*

We've already addressed the sugar issue. Now it's time to look at the others.

Avoid Sedentary Behaviour: Exercise

Real food + exercise = the health miracle we're searching for.

Imagine if there was a pill or potion that could:

- reduce your chance of premature death
- improve your energy levels
- increase aerobic fitness
- build greater muscle strength
- reduce inflammation
- improve balance
- reduce your stress level
- improve your mood
- improve sex performance
- improve brain health and memory
- improve sleep quality
- reduce pain
- improve your blood lipid profile
- improve your immune function
- reduce insulin resistance . . .

while also helping to prevent and/or treat the following chronic diseases:

- **psychiatric diseases**: depression, anxiety, stress, schizophrenia
- **neurological diseases**: dementia, Parkinson's disease, multiple sclerosis
- **metabolic diseases**: obesity, high triglycerides, metabolic syndrome, PCOS, types 1 and 2 diabetes, fatty liver
- **cardiovascular diseases**: high blood pressure, heart disease, heart failure, stroke, intermittent claudication, deep-vein thrombosis (DVT)

- **lung diseases**: chronic obstructive pulmonary disease, asthma, cystic fibrosis
- **musculoskeletal disorders**: osteoarthritis, osteoporosis, back pain, rheumatoid arthritis
- **cancer**.

Wow! How much would you pay for a tablet that did all that? Well, there is one thing that can do all this: EXERCISE.

Why wouldn't you do it then?

The benefits of exercise

There's substantial evidence that exercise can provide benefits for at least 30 chronic diseases. Exercise interventions have been shown to be more effective than drug treatment among patients with stroke, and were as effective as medications for the prevention of diabetes and secondary treatment of cardiovascular disease.[1] Exercise can be as effective as medications for treating depression, and has a positive effect on cognitive function in dementia and Alzheimer's disease.[2]

A review published in 2017 revisited more than 100 studies involving tens of thousands of cancer patients worldwide and found that death rates among those who exercised regularly were 28–44 per cent lower. The risk of cancer recurring was as much as 35 per cent lower, and there were fewer side effects from chemotherapy among those suffering predominantly from breast, bowel and prostate cancer.[3] Other reviews have identified reductions in the risk of most major chronic diseases of 25–50 per cent or more in people who manage 150 minutes of moderate-intensity physical activity a week.[4]

In an eight-year Australian study involving more than 200 000 adults, each 10 minutes of moderate-intensity physical activity per day led to a reduction in the relative risk of death by roughly 10 per cent, which increased to 32–44 per cent with 150 minutes moderate-intensity physical activity per week.[5]

Exercise and weight loss

While exercise has numerous benefits, it only plays a small role in weight loss. As US physician Dr Yoni Freedhoff put it, 'You lose weight in the kitchen, you gain health in the gym.'[6]

There's a belief that you can eat or drink whatever you like because you can 'always run it off'. Even with the now-discredited calories in, calories out theory, it was still virtually impossible to do enough exercise to expend more calories than your intake. The effect of exercise on weight does vary between individuals, and some people are quite sensitive to the effects of exercise, but for most of us, as Tim Noakes, Steve Phinney and Aseem Malhotra put it, 'You can't outrun a bad diet.'[7]

Exercise may be more helpful in *maintaining* weight loss (rather than stimulating it) as found in a study of competitors from *The Biggest Loser*. The study found that *The Biggest Loser* participants who were the most successful in maintaining lost weight had the greatest increase in physical activity after six years.[8]

Physical activity guidelines

Australia's 2014 *Physical Activity and Sedentary Behaviour Guidelines* recommend that adult Australians aged 18–64:

- Be active on most, preferably all, days every week.
- Accumulate 150–300 minutes of moderate-intensity physical activity or 75–150 minutes of vigorous-intensity physical activity, or an equivalent combination of the two, each week.
- Do muscle-strengthening activities on at least two days each week.
- Minimise the amount of time spent in prolonged sitting.
- Break up long periods of sitting as often as possible.

The guidelines recommend that children and young people (aged 5–17) accumulate at least 60 minutes of moderate to vigorous physical activity every day. They also recommend that older Australians (65 years and older) should be active every day in as many ways as possible, and accumulate at least 30 minutes of moderate-intensity physical activity on most and preferably all days.

Are we meeting the guidelines?

Based on self-reported data from the *2014–15 National Health Survey*, 56 per cent of Australian adults didn't participate in sufficient physical activity, and this generally got worse with age as the table shows.

Adults living in regional and remote areas are, on average, more

Insufficient activity among Australian adults

Age group	All adults (%)	Men (%)	Women (%)
18–24	48	45	51
25–34	47	44	49
35–44	53	53	54
45–54	57	57	56
55–64	57	54	60
64+	75	74	77

Source: ABS, *National Health Survey, First Results 2014–15*, 2015[9]

likely to be insufficiently active than those living in major cities, and this increases with socioeconomic disadvantage. In 2014–15, 60 per cent of men and 66 per cent of women living in the most disadvantaged areas were insufficiently active, compared with 38 per cent of men and 43 per cent of women living in the least disadvantaged areas.

According to the Heart Foundation, in 2008 physical inactivity cost the Australian economy $13.8 billion.[10]

Why aren't we exercising?

The main reasons people give are:

1. **Lack of time:** We all lead busy lives, and it's easy to convince ourselves we don't have time for exercise. It's just a matter of priorities.
2. **Lack of motivation:** It often takes a major health scare (e.g. a non-fatal heart attack) to get people concerned enough about their health to start exercising. Surely it's better to take measures to prevent the heart attack in the first place!
3. **Lack of enjoyment/boredom:** It's important to find a type of activity or sport that you enjoy, and will continue to enjoy.
4. **Injury/illness:** You may have an injury or a degenerative condition such as osteoarthritis of the knee that prevents you from doing a specific activity such as running. In that case, try a non-weight bearing activity such as cycling or swimming.

How much exercise we need

Ideally, we'd get our 150 minutes of weekly moderate-intensity exercise by doing 30 minutes, five times per week, of aerobic activities – such as jogging, cycling, swimming or ballroom dancing. Moderate intensity (see the table below) means you're working in the intermediate zone. If you can hold a conversation while doing that activity, you're in that zone. The recommended 30 minutes of exercise a day can be done in one bout or alternatively in a number of different bouts, such as three lots of ten minutes.

As much as 150 minutes a week may seem impossible to sedentary people, but there are measurable benefits with even small amounts of physical activity. The biggest positive change in mortality risk – a drop of 15 per cent – can be achieved simply by going from completely inactive to somewhat active (doing 75–90 minutes of weekly activity).

An alternative to the 150 minutes of moderate-intensity activity is 75 minutes of vigorous aerobic activity a week, which may include such activities as running, swimming, racquet sports and ball games.

The good news: if you don't have time for five workouts a week, doing all of your 150 minutes on the weekend provides similar health benefits. The only risk 'weekend warriors' run here is overuse injury, after doing a sudden burst of activity – such as running 10 kilometres – after no exercise during the week.

Degrees of physical activity

Intensity	Objective measures	What you feel	Typical examples
Sedentary	<1.6 METs <40% HRmax <20% VO2max	At rest with limited added movement	Sitting and reading Watching TV Driving a car
Light	1.6–3.0 METs 40–55% HRmax 20–40% VO2max	Active No noticeable change in breathing/sweating Can be sustained for 1 hour or more	Slow walking (e.g. around the house) Light work while standing (e.g. cooking, washing dishes) Playing an instrument
Moderate	3–6 METs 55–70% HRmax 40–60% VO2max	Increased breathing and sweating, but still able to maintain a conversation Can sustain activity for 30–60 minutes	Brisk walk Low-movement racquet games (e.g. doubles tennis, recreational badminton) Water aerobics Resistance exercise Mowing the lawn

Intensity	Objective measures	What you feel	Typical examples
Vigorous	6–9 METs 70–90% HRmax 60–85% VO2max	Feeling 'out of breath' Increased sweating Can be difficult to maintain a conversation Can sustain activity for up to 30 minutes	Jogging Hiking Swimming with effort Higher-movement racquet games (e.g. singles tennis and squash) Field/ball games (e.g. soccer and basketball) Cross-country skiing Shovelling
High	≥9 METs ≥90% HRmax ≥85% VO2max	Feels like giving 100 per cent All-out bursts of 1–2 minutes Intensity can't be sustained for more than 10 minutes	Training/competing in most competitive sports Racing or any all-out activity (e.g. running, rowing, swimming, skiing and high-intensity intervals in HIIT)

Key: HRmax = theoretical maximal heart rate, usually estimated as (220 − age); MET = metabolic equivalent of task (where 1 MET = the energy to lie or sit quietly); VO2max = maximal oxygen uptake

Source: Thornton, J.S., et al., *Br J Sports Med*, 2016[11]

REDUCE SITTING TIME

Cutting down your time spent sitting is also important. The average office worker spends nine hours a day sitting. The more hours we sit each day, the higher our risk of metabolic problems, even if we achieve the recommended amount of daily physical activity.

Two recent studies, one from Australia and one from the US, found that the total duration of daily inactivity and of each bout of sedentary behaviour were both linked to increased risk of death from any cause, even taking into account age, sex, education, smoking and high blood pressure and moderate to vigorous physical activity.[12]

If you have to work at a desk all day, consider a standing desk, or at least make sure you get up and walk for a couple of minutes about every 30–40 minutes.

Is more exercise better?

The Australian study mentioned above found improvements in mortality with increasing amounts of exercise up to 3–5 times the guidelines (i.e. 450–750 minutes a week), and the reduction in mortality appeared to plateau at 50–60 per cent.

There is a certain amount of exercise beyond which you get no additional health benefit. So if you continue to exercise beyond that, you're doing it for reasons other than your health. Those reasons can be quite valid and could include a specific performance goal, competition, or simply wanting to overcome a personal challenge, such as finishing a marathon or an ironman competition.

The most common mistake made is to increase the amount of activity too quickly. The body responds very well to increased load as long as that increase is gradual – no more than 10 per cent per week. Any more than that and the body will start to show signs of fatigue and injuries may occur.

After strenuous exercise, the body needs time to recover. Recovery involves replacing lost fluid, replacing energy stores and sleep. Sleep is a very important component of recovery.

10 000 steps

It's become a popular mantra that we need 10 000 steps a day. It was introduced because having an easy-to-remember aim can provide the motivation necessary to improve physical activity levels.

If we assume a moderate-intensity walking rhythm of 100 steps per minute, 30 minutes of walking is equal to 3000 steps. As about 5000 steps a day of incidental exercise associated with normal daily living is generally regarded as average, combined with walking for 30 minutes this would give a total of about 8000 steps a day. Fifty minutes of walking would be required to lift the number of steps to 10 000. Alternatively, you could say that 10 000 steps equates to roughly 8 kilometres of walking a day for an average-sized adult.

If aiming for a finite number like 10 000 steps helps you, then go for it. Obviously it doesn't take into account activities such as swimming, cycling, yoga, Pilates and so on, so it's not always an accurate measure of physical activity.

There isn't much research comparing the health benefit of different numbers of steps, although there's some evidence that up to 15 000 steps at least, there seem to be added health benefits. Most health and fitness experts think around 10 000 is about right.

Your exercise regime

The best exercise program combines some aerobic activity, which could be one of:

- 150 minutes a week of moderate activity
- 75 minutes a week of vigorous activity
- your favourite HIIT program (see below)

with a strength-training program (see page 216) twice a week. It might also be worth incorporating some flexibility training, either as a warm-up or cool-down, or as a separate activity.

Exercise tips

1. Enjoy it! It's not important what type of exercise you do, just find one you enjoy. If you don't enjoy it, you won't stick at it.
2. If you're a social animal, find someone or a group to exercise with. It's harder to not turn up for a session if someone else is expecting you.
3. Remember that it doesn't have to be vigorous. A brisk walk is fine.
4. Incorporate walking into your daily routine – leave the car at home, walk to the shops, park some distance from work and walk the rest of the way.
5. Take the stairs or at least a few flights (I don't expect you to walk up to the 53rd floor!).
6. Instead of meeting a friend for coffee, suggest a walk (maybe followed by coffee!).

HIIT

Many of us don't have the time for or get bored with 150 minutes of moderate exercise a week. And even 75 minutes a week of vigorous exercise can be too much of a commitment. If that's your situation, HIT or HIIT – high-intensity interval training – could be the answer.

HIIT involves a number of short bursts of intense exercise followed by rest or reduced exercise. Examples might be sprinting (or cycling/swimming and so on) for 20, 30 or 60 seconds at high intensity, followed by

10 seconds, 30 seconds, 1 minute or 3 minutes of rest or minimal activity such as walking (or gentle cycling, and so on). This can be repeated a number of times.

Popular forms of HIIT include:

- Tabata, which involves 20 seconds of intense activity followed by 10 seconds of recovery, repeated up to 6–8 times. Eight sets would then involve a total of 4 minutes.
- The 'seven-minute workout', which consists of twelve different exercises (e.g. push-ups, crunches, etc.), each performed at high intensity for 30 seconds followed by a 10-second break.
- The 'one-minute workout', which involves a two-minute warm-up, three 20-second flat-out sprints and a three-minute cool down – a total of one minute of high intensity.

There's limited research on the effectiveness of HIIT.[13] Some small studies have shown improvements in risk factors for type 2 diabetes.[14] A larger study published in 2017 incorporating a '5 × 1' program – five bouts of one minute's intense exercise with 90 seconds of recovery between – performed three times a week for six weeks, showed improvements in aerobic fitness, blood pressure and insulin resistance, all of which were maintained three weeks after training stopped.[15]

At this stage we can say these things about HIIT:

1. It seems to provide just as much benefit as the traditional 150 minutes a week of aerobic exercise.
2. There's no evidence that one type of HIIT is better than any other. All the different regimes have a similar positive effect.
3. We don't really know how often you should do HIIT – most suggest 2–3 times a week, but once a week has been recommended by some.
4. It all comes down to factors like time availability and individual preferences.

The secret of HIIT seems to be not the energy you expend during the workout itself, but the post-workout increase in metabolic rate. Because it doesn't really matter what type of exercise you do, it's easy to incorporate HIIT into your daily activity. Intense stair climbing for 20, 30 or 60 seconds is one simple way. I know someone who, when watching his favourite

TV show, stands up in each ad break and does 20 seconds of intense activity, such as high-knee running on the spot or push-ups.

Resistance exercise

Before you skip this section thinking it is only about pumping iron and being a gym junkie, think again. Everyone should be doing some strength training, particularly as you get older.

Growing older, we face entering a physical decline that will reduce our ability to walk, carry shopping, and complete other very simple tasks that we all normally take for granted when younger. One of the main issues as we get older is loss of muscle mass and bone density. This leads to an increased incidence of falls and fractures, which can often begin a rapid deterioration in the health of an older person.

Unless we do something about it, the average person will lose muscle mass at a rate of around 8 per cent per decade, but after the age of 70 years, the rate of this loss rises to 15 per cent per decade. This loss of muscle mass translates into substantially reduced strength, which is particularly important for mobility. Increased muscle strength positively correlates with an increased functional ability as we age. We need muscle power for many daily living activities, such as getting out of a chair, walking up stairs and lifting things. Improving strength has been shown to also improve balance. Muscular strength and muscle mass are predictors of longevity.[16]

There's also evidence that resistance training decreases gastrointestinal transit time (reducing the risk of colon cancer), increases metabolic rate, reduces lower-back pain, increases bone mineral density, reduces blood pressure, and improves muscle quality and insulin sensitivity in people with type 2 diabetes.[17]

You don't have to spend hours in the gym to get the beneficial effect. It seems that as few as three gym exercises using multiple joints (e.g. chest press, leg press, seated row) with resistance that leads to muscle fatigue at 8–12 reps separated by 90 seconds, can provide positive benefits with a total workout time of less than 10 minutes. If you do that twice a week you'll get significant health benefits for 20 minutes of effort a week. Good value!

You don't even need to go to the gym. Simple exercises like squats just using body weight can be very helpful in the elderly. Everyday activities like carrying shopping bags and walking up stairs are actually strength training activities.

Flexibility

Stretching is often promoted as having a number of beneficial effects, such as increased muscle and joint flexibility, increased muscle relaxation, decreased muscle soreness and improved circulation, but not all of these have been appropriately studied. Traditionally, stretching has been recommended to prevent injury and enhance performance for sporting activity. Some authors have suggested, however, that stretching does not prevent injury in otherwise healthy individuals.[18]

Stretching can be performed immediately before exercise, after exercise as part of a warm-down, or as part of a general conditioning program. Each muscle probably has its ideal length, and there's no point trying to stretch it beyond that. Stretching is useful, though, for overcoming stiff, tight muscles and restoring them to their normal length.

Stretching can be static or dynamic. It was thought that dynamic warm-ups were risky, but as long as the dynamic stretches aren't performed on cold muscles they're fine. In fact, most professional sporting teams incorporate dynamic stretching into their warm-ups once the muscle is warm.

My exercise routine

I'm pretty time-poor and also get bored by monotonous aerobic exercise, so I've been doing my own version of HIIT for the past few years on a stationary exercise bike. I have a nine-minute program that consists of:

- a two-minute warm-up
- four intervals of 30 seconds' flat-out cycling, with 30 seconds of easy pedalling between (four minutes in total)
- four intervals of 15 seconds' flat-out cycling, with 15 seconds of easy pedalling between (two minutes in total)
- a one-minute warm-down.

In reality, I'm doing a total of three minutes' intense exercise in a nine-minute program.

I then do some strength training, usually with dumbbells or, if I'm on the road, whatever equipment the hotel gym has. If I'm away from any equipment, I do a session with push-ups, abdominal crunches and single-leg squats.

I like the single-leg squat as an exercise because it works your lower limb, your glutes and your core, and is also a good balance exercise. You can do it anywhere. I often do it when I'm waiting around for something (I get a few strange looks!).

POINTS TO REMEMBER
- Exercise has clear health benefits and Australian guidelines recommend 150 minutes a week of aerobic activity.
- High intensity interval training (HIIT) is an alternative for those who are time-poor.
- Resistance training can help maintain muscle strength as we age.

Achieve More
Good-quality Sleep

Without good sleep, good health is impossible.

Recent research from the Sleep Health Foundation suggests that about 40 per cent of us are getting poor-quality sleep or not sleeping long enough – 10 per cent say they're sleeping less than five and a half hours a night – which is making us tired and cranky. A third of people said tiredness had made them make mistakes, and 20 per cent had drifted off while driving. Women generally have more trouble than men falling asleep, and then wake up too early feeling unrefreshed. Even when they get as many hours of sleep as men, they don't feel replenished by sleep.[1]

Why sleep is important

Poor sleep can rapidly undermine our efforts to improve our health and our weight. This is because it affects the hormones involved in making us hungry and storing fat.

During deep sleep, the pituitary gland normally releases growth hormone, lack of which can help accelerate premature ageing. We need deep sleep to replace and repair muscle and bone, and to consolidate neurological function, which makes it the most important factor in recovery from intense exercise and competition, allowing the body to recover in time for the next training session. Good sleep is also important for cognitive function, laying down memories and motor learning.

What happens if we don't get enough sleep

The repercussions of lack of sleep are now showing up around our waistlines and in our overall poor health.

Obesity

Summaries of research have shown a link between reduced length of sleep and obesity.[2] In studies of children aged three to five, each additional hour of sleep per night was associated with a 61 per cent reduction in the risk of being overweight or obese by the age of seven.[3] One study linked a single extra hour of sleep a night to a 28 per cent lower risk of being overweight and a 30 per cent lower risk of obesity.[4]

Sleep length has a direct impact on two hunger-related hormones, ghrelin and leptin. The less we sleep, the higher the ghrelin, the lower the leptin levels and the hungrier we are.[5]

Limited sleep (about four hours a night) has been shown to make people eat more than after a full night's rest.[6] Lack of sleep can slow the metabolism and is linked with insulin resistance – both of which contribute to obesity.[7]

Insulin resistance and type 2 diabetes

When young healthy men are sleep deprived, they have higher fasting insulin levels. Just one night of sleep deprivation can lead to similar disruptions in insulin sensitivity to six months of unhealthy eating. Lack of sleep is also associated with increased inflammation, which can also lead to higher insulin levels.[8]

Glucose metabolism can be seriously affected by even short-term changes in sleep. Sleep deprivation lasting one to five days leads to impaired glucose levels. One study followed 1455 adults for six years and found that fasting glucose levels were significantly higher in those who slept less than six hours a night.[9]

In another study, a single night of sleep reduction from eight to four hours reduced the rate of uptake of glucose from the blood by 25 per cent.[10]

Impaired brain function

Insufficient sleep can impair memory. Even one night of four to six hours' sleep can affect our ability to think clearly the following day. It can also reduce our performance in mental and physical tasks, and affect problem-solving.[11]

Too little sleep is a risk factor for Alzheimer's disease, and continued lack of sleep can hasten its progression. People with regular poor sleep had more plaques in their brains. The researchers theorised that sleep is vital for ridding us of 'cerebral waste', and that habitual poor sleep allows it to accumulate, leading to dementia.[12]

Cardiovascular disease

Lack of sleep can result in raised blood pressure and increased risk of heart disease. In a long-term Russian study of men aged 25–64, almost two-thirds of those who suffered heart attacks also had sleep disorders. The men with sleep disorders also had a much greater risk of myocardial infarction and stroke.[13]

Inflammation and chronic diseases

Getting less than seven to eight hours of sleep per night can result in increased levels of inflammatory markers such as CRP in the blood. These markers have been linked to chronic conditions such as cardiovascular disease, high blood pressure and type 2 diabetes, which suggests that poor sleep is as much of a risk factor for inflammation as a poor diet or sedentary lifestyle.[14]

According to a study conducted by the NHS in the United Kingdom, less than six hours' sleep (or, interestingly enough, more than nine) can trigger ulcerative colitis, an inflammatory bowel disease that causes ulcers in the lining of the digestive tract.[15]

Mental illness

When we don't sleep well, we can quickly blow things out of proportion, overreacting to neutral events, feeling provoked for no reason, and being unable to determine what's important, which can result in poor judgement and bias.

Lack of sleep increases the risk of depression. In one trial with depressed people, 87 per cent of those who were able to overcome their insomnia experienced major improvements in mood, and their symptoms disappeared after eight weeks.[16] A 2014 study from Stanford University found a link between a lack of sleep and suicidal thoughts in adults, even among those hadn't reported feeling depressed before.[17]

Lack of sleep also appears to worsen behavioural difficulties in children.[18] Most parents would agree with that statement!

Cancer

There have been suggestions that lack of sleep may make people more susceptible to developing cancer. One three-year study from Iceland, which examined more than 2000 men aged 67–96, found that those who had inadequate sleep were 60 per cent more likely to develop prostate cancer. The researchers that this was a result of suppression of the sleep hormone melatonin, since melatonin both allows for better sleep quality and represses tumor growth.[19]

Night shiftwork on only three nights a month is associated with a higher rate of cancer, and the risk increases with more shiftwork.[20] People who do shiftwork have disrupted circadian rhythm and melatonin secretion, which leads to increased rates of anxiety, depression, chronic fatigue, ulcers and cardiovascular disease.

Pain and injury

Lack of sleep can aggravate chronic pain. In one study in adults over 50, poor or insufficient sleep was the strongest predictor of pain.

There is also evidence lack of sleep can lead to injury. Teenage athletes who sleep less than eight hours a night had a 1.7 times higher risk of injury risk than those sleeping eight or more hours.[21] Another study found that young runners and soccer, basketball and gridiron players who slept six hours or less a night experienced more fatigue-related injuries.[22]

How much sleep do we need?

If you leap out of bed each morning alert and ready to face the day, you're getting enough sleep. If you're lethargic and tired during the day, you probably need more. Our sleep needs vary from person to person, and depend on things like age and health.

The American National Sleep Foundation recommends seven to nine hours per night for adults, but length of sleep on its own isn't enough – the sleep needs to be of good quality and when we need it. Going to sleep and waking up at similar times each day is also useful. Don't fall for the trap of going to bed early if you didn't sleep well the night before.

When we get less than seven hours' sleep we don't perform at our best. When we habitually get less than six hours' sleep a night, our risk of health problems increases.

How to get a good night's sleep

There's no one magic ingredient to getting a good night's sleep. Everyone's different. You can do a few things to help though, during the day, in the evening and before you go to bed. I hope some or all of the following measures will help. If not, it might be time for some professional help.

During the day

- **Get natural sunlight**: When you wake up and it's already light, open the curtains. Exposure to bright light first thing in the morning stops production of the sleep-inducing hormone melatonin and signals to your body that it's time to wake up. Outdoor sunlight is best, so you might even want to take a 15–20 minute walk outside. Then, around the middle of the day, get another 'dose' of at least 30 minutes' worth of sunlight. A full hour or more would be even better. If your schedule means you have to get up and arrive at work before sunrise, aim to get at least that half-hour of bright sunlight sometime during the day. Tweaking these exposures to bright natural light in the morning and no exposure to blue light at night is critical to healthy sleep. At night, as the sun sets, darkness should signal to your body that it's time to sleep.
- **Make your bed**: This is a psychological trick aimed at making your bedroom less cluttered, and therefore easier to relax in come bedtime.
- **Exercise**: Exercise leads to better sleep at night. It doesn't have to be a big workout to enjoy sleep benefits. If the exercise is outside in the sunshine, that's even better.

In the evening

- **Avoid excess alcohol**: I find that more than one or two drinks a night impairs the quality of my sleep.
- **Watch your evening meal**: Eat a light dinner and stop eating three hours before bedtime. Avoid spicy foods, steak and citrus fruits. Eat foods high in melatonin (miso, cherries, salmon) and tryptophan (milk, bananas).
- **Curtail the caffeine**: Avoid coffee and caffeinated drinks after mid-afternoon.
- **Have a calming tea**: Drink a herbal tea containing lavender, valerian, passionflower or chamomile to soothe and calm the nervous system.

Before you go to bed

- Stick to a regular schedule: Try to have a regular bedtime and a regular routine before you go to bed.

- Reduce light exposure: No artificial bright lights or TV in the bedroom, and avoid using your phone, tablet or laptop in bed.
- Avoid the need to pee during the night: Don't drink any fluids within two hours of going to bed and go to the toilet right before bed.
- Avoid before-bed snacks: Particularly grains, sugars and any caffeinated drinks.
- Try to unwind mentally: Put your work away at least one hour before bed and take 15 minutes to unwind. Meditation can be very helpful.

During the night

- **Watch the room temperature**: Keep the temperature in your bedroom no higher than 21°C. Use light bedclothes or sleep naked.
- **Try sex**: We blokes are always accused of falling asleep straight after sex, so why not use that to help you sleep!
- **Consider separate bedrooms**: If your partner is a restless or noisy sleeper, this might be worth a try.
- **Keep it dark**: Sleep in complete darkness or as close to it as possible. Even the tiniest bit of light in the room can disrupt your internal clock and production of melatonin. Close your bedroom door, get rid of night-lights, cover up your clock radio, cover your windows (use blackout if necessary) and/or wear an eye mask to block out light.

Some people desperate for sleep go to great lengths to avoid exposure to blue light in the evening before bed, wearing amber-coloured glasses that block blue light, using low-wattage bulbs with light at the red end of the spectrum, and installing blue-light-blocking software on their devices. There are also lots of simple suggestions that work for individual people, such as moving electrical devices away from the bed, taking a hot bath before bed or writing in a daily journal.

Being overweight can increase the risk of sleep apnoea (see page 227), which can make quality sleep impossible, so losing weight can have a big impact on sleep.

Finally, try not to get too anxious about not sleeping. The more anxious you are, the less likely you are to sleep. Rest is nearly as beneficial as sleep, though, so if you can rest without sleeping you're still getting some benefit.

SLEEPING PILLS

Many people see sleeping tablets as the solution to either difficulty getting to sleep, or difficulty staying asleep. These can be pharmaceuticals such as benzodiazepines and benzodiazepine receptor agonists, or over-the-counter herbal supplements, such as valerian, hops, passionflower and kava kava.

Sleeping tablets can be useful for short-term use in specific situations – before an exam, job interview, surgery or sporting event. They can also be useful in managing jet lag (see below). It's important to be aware of these facts and guidelines for sleeping tablets:

- They can cause dependence, so only use them in the short term (up to four weeks).
- Don't mix them with alcohol.
- Be careful when taking other medications (check with your GP).
- The side effects can include excessive fatigue, unsteadiness and vivid dreams.
- They usually work within 15–30 minutes but become less effective over time.

Jet lag

Jet lag occurs when the body can't adapt rapidly enough to a time-zone shift and normal body rhythms get out of sync. The main problems associated with jet lag are daytime fatigue, poor sleep and impaired performance.

Australians do a lot of long distance international travel, more than any other nationality, and jet lag is a major problem. There is nothing worse than sitting in a meeting or a conference in the United States or Europe with an overwhelming urge to close your eyes and nod off.

I've been travelling to conferences and with sporting teams now for more than 30 years, and while I'm much better than I used to be, I still occasionally get hit by a bad case of jet lag. Of course, it can be just as bad on the return leg, so when you're back home catching up with work or family, you can have that same sense of fatigue.

It's always been said that it takes a day per time zone crossed for the biological clock to resynchronise with the sleep–wake cycle. If you're travelling to the West Coast of the United States, for instance, that means it would be two weeks before you were functioning normally again. Fortunately, we can usually do better than that.

It's probably impossible to completely eliminate jet lag, but you can do a few things to help you function better after a long plane trip.

Pre-departure

Is there anything you can do before departure to reduce the impact of jet lag on arrival? There's been much discussion about changing to the arrival country's time zone in the few days before you leave. That's a good idea in theory, but unrealistic – in practice it's extremely difficult, assuming you have to work before you go.

During the flight

Australians generally have a 14–16-hour flight to the United States or a 22–24-hour flight with one stopover to Europe. Assuming you can sleep on the flight (which many people can't), the first thing to do is to work out the best time to sleep. For that, it's best to work backwards from your arrival time.

If you're arriving in the morning, try to delay your sleep until the hours before arriving. If, on the other hand, you're arriving late afternoon or evening, try to sleep during the first part of the flight and stay awake in the hours before arrival. That way, when you get there, you can get to your accommodation, have something to eat and then be ready for bed at the (new) normal time.

That sleeping schedule can be difficult if, for example, you're departing at night after a busy day, and you want to try and stay awake for the first part of a journey with a morning arrival, but it's worth a try. In a situation like that, a short initial sleep followed by a period awake and then another sleep before your early morning arrival might work well.

There are a few things you can do on the plane to help minimise the effect of jet lag. Avoid excess food and/or alcohol. By all means have a drink, especially before sleep time, but avoid the temptation to overdo it if there's free booze. It's also easy to overeat on a flight, so I usually try to skip at least one of the meals in a 24-hour period.

On arrival

The keys to overcoming jet lag are sunshine, exercise and sleep. Your body needs to be made aware that it needs to change its sleep–wake cycle. The best stimulus for that is exposure to sunlight, so if you arrive in the morning and want to stay awake until bedtime, then the more exposure to sunlight you get, the better. Try to resist the temptation to stay in your hotel room (and fall asleep), and get outside. Exercise in the sun is even better, so a long walk, run or cycle will help. Caffeine can help stave off fatigue as well.

If you find it absolutely impossible to stay awake, allow yourself a short nap, but keep it to one hour max, set an alarm to wake yourself up, and get outside into the sunshine.

Sleep

If you've made it through until bedtime, well done. But that doesn't automatically mean you'll have a full night's sleep. Your body clock is still confused and taking time to adjust. I often find that the first night's sleep is good (and I congratulate myself that I have sorted out this jet lag thing once and for all), only to have a shocker the second (and subsequent) night.

It's awful to wake up in a foreign hotel room, feeling wide awake, knowing there's no way you'll be able to get back to sleep, only to look over at the clock and find it's 2 a.m. and you've been asleep for a mere three or four hours. You can always try to get back to sleep or use any of the tricks mentioned above, but sometimes you know in your heart of hearts you won't be able to.

Those situations are the only times I ever use a sleeping tablet. I have a 4 a.m. rule: if I wake up before 4 a.m. and know I am not going to be able to get back to sleep by myself, I take one of the short-acting sleeping tablets e.g. Imovane, which will usually give me another four hours' sleep. If I wake up after 4 a.m., I just get up and get going – there are always emails to be handled, presentations to prepare, or newspapers/journal articles to be read.

Sleep apnoea

Obstructive sleep apnoea (OSA) is a chronic disease where the airway repeatedly becomes blocked during sleep, resulting in reduced oxygen availability and recurrent waking. It's common in Western society, affecting about 2 per cent of women and 4 per cent of men.[23]

Obesity is the strongest risk factor for developing OSA. It has been estimated that 58 per cent of moderate to severe OSA is due to obesity. Obesity acts directly to narrow the airway through an increase in neck circumference and fat deposits around the airway itself. The upper airway is also more prone to collapse in obese people, and their lung volume is higher. Nerve and muscle response in the upper airway is also blunted by abdominal fat.

Men are two to three times more likely to develop OSA. This increased risk could be related to the way fat is distributed in men. Increases in abdominal fat with age could also explain the increase in OSA among middle-aged and older men and postmenopausal women.

OSA also leads to increased obesity, setting up a vicious cycle of increased weight and worsening OSA. It's not clear what causes this effect, but as we've seen, sleep deprivation can lead to obesity, and although people with sleep apnoea may feel like they've been asleep all night, they won't feel rested.

There's plenty of evidence that weight loss reduces the occurrence of OSA. A decrease in weight of as little as 10 per cent can improve the severity of OSA.[24]

It's also been suggested that treating the underlying sleep problem may be effective in managing obesity. Successful treatment of sleep apnoea, usually with nasal continuous positive airway pressure (CPAP) can reduce sleepiness, which motivates weight loss, helping with both obesity and OSA.[25]

Snoring

Heavy snoring can be associated with OSA, but it's often an isolated symptom. As with OSA there's a link between snoring and obesity due to the excess of fat around the neck causing narrowing of the upper airway. Other risk factors for snoring are alcohol consumption (due to muscle relaxation), taking sedatives, smoking and hay fever.[26]

My sleeping habits

Before I lost weight by making changes to the way I eat, I was a big snorer, and probably had mild OSA. It was just one of the many things about me that used to drive my wife mad! At least now there is one less thing – I no longer snore. I've also noticed that I'm much less sleepy in the afternoon, which has helped me spend 14 hours a day writing this damn book!

POINTS TO REMEMBER

- About 40 per cent of us have either poor quality or poor quantity of sleep. Poor sleep is associated with numerous health issues.
- There are numerous tricks to help increase sleep.
- Sleep apnoea is a common condition closely related to obesity.

Reduce Stress

Stress can lead to chronic inflammation and any number
of health conditions.

Stress is inescapable, but how you deal with it is what determines whether it causes health problems. This ability of the body to deal with stress is called resilience – 'the ability of your body to rapidly return to normal, both physically and emotionally, after a stressful event'. Some people are naturally more resilient than others, and researchers have long pondered the reasons why.

How stress affects the body

When we're in a stressful situation, real or imagined, our body releases cortisol and other stress hormones so that we can either fight or flee. We all know the feeling: our heart beats faster, we breathe more quickly to take in more oxygen, and we can feel the blood flowing through us. While these physical signs are happening, parts of our immune system are temporarily suppressed, reducing our inflammatory response to disease-causing organisms and other foreign invaders. People who regularly have higher levels of cortisol die younger and are at greater risk of developing cardiovascular disease, type 2 diabetes, metabolic syndrome and other disorders.[1]

In someone who is chronically stressed, the immune system responds less and less to the high cortisol levels. One of the jobs cortisol does is help regulate inflammation, so when the body becomes desensitised to cortisol, the inflammatory response increases and inflammation gets out of control. Inflammation, as we have seen, is a hallmark of most diseases, from type 2 diabetes to cardiovascular disease, cancer and Alzheimer's disease.

Links have been found between stress and numerous conditions, including physical pain, chronic inflammation, stillbirths and an unhealthy gut.[2] Associations have also been seen between stress and cancer susceptibility, survival rates and tumour growth. Stress is also known to cause high blood pressure, and increases the likelihood of developing cardiovascular disease and stroke. Chronic stress at a high level is linked with mood changes, including anger, anxiety, frustration, depression, lack of focus and poor energy. It can have a negative impact on personal relationships and marriages.

Gaining weight and/or having trouble losing it, is commonly associated with stress. When we feel stressed or threatened, our cortisol levels increase the signal to our livers to release more glucose, to provide the fuel to fight or run for our lives. Too much cortisol means too much glucose in our bloodstream and tissues, and any excess will be stored as fat. This kind of weight gain usually occurs by laying down abdominal fat, the most dangerous kind of fat, as it increases the risk of cardiovascular disease. Stress also influences the food we eat, making us choose poor-quality 'comfort' foods.

A recent UK study involving a large group of people over 50 showed that increased waist circumference and body mass index (BMI) were associated with increased cortisol levels in hair, indicating chronic stress.[3]

What causes stress?

Here are a few of the most common stressors in society today:

- anxiety about an upcoming task
- driving, especially being stuck in traffic
- relationship difficulties and divorce
- exams and other milestone tests
- money worries
- grief
- poor health – our own or a family member's
- weight problems
- loneliness
- work problems or unemployment.

Techniques for reducing stress

Whether the stress is at work or in your personal life, your response to it is what matters. To manage stress, you need to know what's causing it and how to deal with it. Here are some of the strategies people use to do this:

- **Get better sleep:** Sleep deprivation dramatically impairs the body's ability to handle stress and is a risk factor for heart attack.

- **Find relaxation and fun time:** Walk in the park, listen to music or play with your children or pets.
- **Do regular physical activity:** Exercising several times a week is great for overall health and a big help in reducing stress.
- **Meditation:** Taking even 10 minutes to sit quietly can help decrease your feelings of stress and anxiety. Try it during work breaks, for example.
- **Do mindfulness training:** See below.
- **Get into yoga:** Regular yoga has been shown to decrease stress, improve sleep and immune function, and reduce food cravings, among other things.[4]
- **Develop social connectedness:** Maintaining good relationships with friends and family can help you stay grounded and give you support when you need it.
- **Confide in someone:** Talking to someone about problems in your life can help you feel better.
- **Keep a diary or journal:** If you don't want to share your feelings with someone else, writing them down in a journal can help.
- **Laugh.**
- **Spend time in nature.**
- **Listen to music.**
- **Find your purpose:** We want to feel like we're achieving something. It can be for a greater good or simply helping someone or feeding your children.
- **Declutter:** Getting rid of unwanted possessions can be liberating.
- **Learn to say no:** You don't have to say yes to everything.
- **Have something to look forward to.**
- **Be grateful for the things you do have:** Try to do this rather than complain about things you don't have.
- **Maintain intimacy with your partner:** There's evidence that physical intimacy can lower stress levels, while a lack of it is associated with feelings of depression and low self-worth.
- **Eat well:** Eat real food. Avoid sugar, processed foods and vegetable oils.

CATHY FREEMAN UNDER EXTREME STRESS

Elite sportspeople operate in a very stressful environment with high public scrutiny and pressure to perform. They develop various techniques to cope.

One of the best examples I've witnessed was Cathy Freeman, Australia's 400 metre gold medallist at the Sydney Olympics. I don't think in the history of the Olympic Games there has ever been a competitor under as much pressure as Cathy. Leading into the Olympics there was a huge media and public focus on her and the expectation of her success. She was our best gold-medal chance in the glamour sport of the Olympics. The night of the 400 metre final was being referred to as 'Freeman night' well before that dramatic evening in Sydney. And then, just in case anyone wasn't aware that Cathy was the star of the show, she was invited to light the Olympic flame in the Opening Ceremony. The whole country was watching and desperately hoping she would win.

And win she did. Not in her best time ever, but not far off it, and good enough to win comfortably in the end. Her reaction when she crossed the finish line was interesting. No wild celebrations – Cathy just sat down on the track with her head in her hands for what seemed to those of us watching an eternity. Then she got up and slowly made her way around the stadium for a lap of honour.

As manager of the Australian Track and Field team in Sydney, one of my tasks was to look after Cathy after her event while she did the rounds of the media, met up with her jubilant family, and had her drug test. We ended up being together for about three hours. Not once in that time did she say how happy she was, how excited she was to have fulfilled her dream. All she said to me time and again was, 'Doc, I'm so relieved . . . Doc, it's such a relief.' No joy, just relief. Relief that she hadn't mucked it up and let herself, her family and her country down. It really drove home to me that night the pressure she'd been under.

Cathy's way of coping with the stress was to tune out. She would withdraw into herself, seemingly oblivious to what was going on around her. That technique certainly held her in good stead in the lead-up to Sydney. It enabled her to avoid much of the hysteria that was going on around her, and allowed her to focus on the job at hand. I'm sure it played a major part in her success. I'm not sure too many other athletes would have coped with the amount of pressure Cathy was under.

Mindfulness and meditation

Mindfulness practice has become a popular pursuit. Classes, books, magazines, blogs and apps are widely available.

It's very easy to get caught up in our thoughts and emotions when we're anxious and stressed. Meditation helps us cut through all that noise so we can deal directly with our stress and listen more attentively to other people and ourselves. The more meditation becomes a habit, the greater the peaceful changes in the mind.

Mindfulness means paying attention to the present moment in a non-judgemental way, while being aware of your body and mind. We can improve mindfulness through meditation exercises that focus on our bodily sensations, breathing or how our thoughts drift through our mind.

Mindfulness meditation is a form of non-religious meditation that draws on aspects of Buddhist meditation. Meditation was traditionally seen as a way to reach enlightenment through liberation from the cycles of life and rebirth. Mindfulness meditation, however, focuses purely on the health benefits of meditation on the brain and body, and, by extension, relationships and everyday life.

When we meditate, our body goes into a physiological state known as the 'relaxation response', a calm feeling of wellbeing.[5] In this state, our blood pressure and cortisol levels drop, and gene expression in our brains is altered. The good thing about the relaxation response is that the changes persist beyond the time of meditation. Regular relaxation through meditation can make a significant difference to our stress levels and wellbeing.

Studies have shown that learning to meditate can increase stem cell production, change hormone responses and reduce inflammation. There is evidence that mindfulness-based programs can reduce anxiety, depression and stress, and help people cope with illness and pain. Some studies show that mindfulness increases positive moods and cultivates compassion. It may also improve some forms of attention and memory.[6]

Practising mindfulness

Mindfulness can be practised in a number of different ways at different levels of intensity:

- **Low-intensity mindfulness**: This is can be done in classes with a teacher leading the session or with self-help books, downloadable recordings or apps. This is the way to get started, and if you find mindfulness really works for you, you might want to increase the intensity of your mindfulness practice.
- **Moderate-intensity mindfulness**: This is used in mindfulness-based stress reduction and cognitive therapy, and other evidence-based mindfulness programs. Typical programs last about eight weeks and involve mindfulness sessions with other participants for up to 40 minutes each day. Although difficult or unwanted memories and emotions can arise during these sessions, they can provide substantial improvements in mental health and wellbeing. These sessions will be followed by discussion with a mindfulness teacher, to make sense of what occurred during the exercise.
- **High-intensity mindfulness**: Meditation retreats provide the most intensive way to practise mindfulness. Participants meditate for many hours each day over the period of a week or more, often entirely in silence. They might have contact with a teacher only once a day or two.

Some of the more popular mindfulness apps are listed on my website, fatlotofgood.com.au.

POINTS TO REMEMBER
- Stress is a part of life – it's how you handle it that matters.
- Stress is related to numerous health problems.
- There are many techniques to improve how we cope with stress, including meditation.

Get Moderate Sun Exposure

We all need some sun to get enough vitamin D.

Have you heard either of these statements?

- Sun is bad for you. Australia has the highest skin cancer rates in the world.
- Sun is good for you. It's the best way to get adequate vitamin D.

Confused? I don't blame you.

Australia used to be a nation of sun-worshippers. We couldn't get enough sun, and a summer suntan was the ultimate status symbol.

Then in 1981, in response to the high incidence of skin cancer in this country, the Cancer Council launched the 'Slip, Slop, Slap' campaign, to encourage the public to *slip* on a shirt, *slop* on sunscreen, and *slap* on a hat. This campaign has been incredibly successful and has resulted in widespread fear of sun. Recently it has been extended to 'Slip, Slop, Slap, Seek and Slide', adding seeking shade and sliding on sunnies to the mix.

Simply put, UVB radiation from the sun is both the best source of vitamin D and the major cause of skin cancer. So we're left wondering whether we should avoid the sun or expose ourselves to it.

The risks of sun exposure: cancer

Skin cancers are of two different types:

1. **Non-melanoma skin cancers (SCC and BCC):** These are the most common malignancies in a pale-skinned older population, but they have an extremely low mortality rate.
2. **Melanomas:** These are much less common, but can spread rapidly and may be fatal.

There's considerable debate about the link between sun and skin cancers, but there's one thing everyone agrees on – getting *sunburnt* is a definite risk factor for all types of skin cancer, including melanoma. So avoid getting burnt at all costs.

After that it gets tricky. The risk of melanoma is increased (by a factor of 1.6) by high levels of intermittent sun exposure, and probably even more by artificial tanning. Artificial UV exposure clearly increases risk for both melanoma and non-melanoma skin cancer, but chronic sun exposure *doesn't* increase the risk of melanoma.[1]

My interpretation of that research is that if you're chronically exposed to sun by working outdoors, you're unlikely to develop melanoma, while if you expose yourself to high levels of sun during your summer beach holiday but spend the rest of the year indoors, you may be at risk.

There is some interesting emerging evidence of a link between diet and melanoma. Specifically, omega-3 fats appear have a protective effect, while omega-6 fats from vegetable oils make our skin more susceptible to UV damage.[2]

The benefits of sun exposure: general health and vitamin D

The first and pretty important thing to note is that overall sun exposure is associated with a reduction in the chance of illness and early death. People who have more exposure to sunlight tend to live longer, even though they tend in general to get more skin cancer.

The benefits of sun exposure can be divided into direct benefits and those associated with vitamin D.

Direct benefits of sun exposure

Exposure to sun is associated with a lower incidence of cardiovascular disease. This could be because when our skin is exposed to the sun, nitric oxide is released into our blood vessels and this lowers blood pressure by causing the blood vessels to dilate.

Increased UV exposure protects from disease by affecting the responses of our hormones, immune system and DNA repair mechanism. It also has therapeutic effects for skin conditions such as psoriasis, eczema and vitiligo. There is also relatively strong evidence that UV exposure can provide a benefit with autoimmune diseases.[3]

Ecological studies have shown that multiple sclerosis (MS) is generally more common the nearer we are to the poles (i.e. at higher lati-tudes), where UV exposure is lowest. Analytical studies demonstrate that higher overall UV exposure is associated with lower rates of MS.[4] Type 1 diabetes also occurs more frequently at higher latitudes.

Nearsightedness is on the rise and that currently affects about 1.5 bil-lion people worldwide. Research has shown the more time spent outdoors, the lower the risk of nearsightedness.[5]

As we have seen numerous times now, inflammation shares strong links with the vast majority of chronic diseases. Regular exposure to UV rays dampens the inflammation response. For this reason, getting suffi-cient sunlight helps reduce chronic disease risk by putting the body in a less inflammatory state.

INDOOR TANNING

In most Westernised countries, particularly in northern Europe and the United States, tanning salons are very popular, and their rates of use are increasing. The International Agency for Research on Cancer concluded that there was a causal link between skin cancer and exposure to both the sun and tanning devices. The strongest evidence for a link between exposure to artificial UV and melanoma is found among people who had their first exposure to indoor tanning before the age of 30: they have a 75 per cent increased risk of developing mela-noma than individuals who had no exposure to indoor tanning.[6]

All this evidence has encouraged many countries to introduce regulations on sunbed use to avoid exposure before the age of 18.

The benefits of vitamin D

Vitamin D plays a role in every system in the body, affecting our skin, brain health, bones, blood sugar, cholesterol, hormone balance, joint health, risk for cancer, and likelihood of developing autoimmune disease.

Vitamin D is unique in that it's not used in the body like most vitamins. It's actually better classified as a hormone. Its primary role in the body is to maintain normal blood levels of calcium and phosphorus, but it has far-reaching effects across body systems – bones, cardiovascular, endocrine, neural function, immune health, and a whole lot more. Vitamin D regulates the activity of over 200 genes, which is many more than any other vitamin.

There's considerable controversy about the importance of vitamin D. Opinions range from considering it 'fairly irrelevant' to 'the most important influence on health'. As usual, the truth is probably somewhere in between. There is some evidence to suggest that vitamin D has the following effects:[7]

- Deficiency results in inadequate mineralisation or demineralisation of the bones, which in children can lead to rickets, causing bowed legs and knocked knees, and in adults can lead to increased bone turnover and osteoporosis.
- Adequate levels are associated with reduced all-cause mortality.
- Adequate levels may reduce the number of falls in the elderly.
- Adequate levels may reduce the incidence of colorectal and breast cancer.
- Adequate levels protect against age-related macular degeneration.
- Adequate levels have the same effect on depression as antidepressants.
- It is significantly related to all types of dementia, including Alzheimer's disease.
- Diabetics have lower vitamin D levels, and all-cause mortality is higher in diabetics with the lowest vitamin D levels.
- Neurodegenerative diseases like Parkinson's occurs less frequently in people with the highest vitamin D levels (67 per cent lower risk).
- Low levels in pregnant women, who are especially at risk of vitamin D deficiency, are associated with increased risk of premature birth.

It has long been suggested that low vitamin D levels may be associated with an increase in colds and flu in the winter. Recent research from Queen Mary Hospital in London seems to confirm that relationship: their results show 10 per cent reduction in cold and flu rates among everyone who takes vitamin D every day or once a week.[8] But the benefit is more pronounced among those who start with low levels of vitamin D in their system, halving the rate of these infections.

A Swedish study showed the mortality rate amongst avoiders of sun exposure was approximately twofold higher compared with the highest sun exposure group.[9] Another study demonstrated that low levels of vitamin D are associated with higher rates of death from all causes and from cardiovascular disease, as the graph below shows.

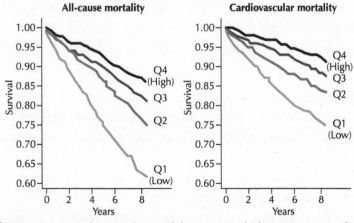

Graph comparing survival rates in those with lowest (01) to highest (04) quarters of vitamin D levels. Those with highest levels have a dramatically reduced all-cause mortality and mortality from cardiovascular disease. *Source:* Dobnig, H., et al., *Arch Intern Med*, 2008[10]

Vitamin D and the sun

Until the past couple of decades, vitamin D deficiency was thought to be extremely rare in Australia. After all, we have high levels of sunlight for most of the year in most of the country. And yet, probably because of our 'sun fear', we've significantly reduced our sun exposure and the latest Australian Health Survey showed that one in four Australian adults are vitamin D deficient, with the highest rates of deficiency in the southern states.

Vitamin D is made in the skin when we're exposed to UVB light at a very specific wavelength. The UVB rays interact with a precursor in the skin, 7-dehydrocholesterol, turning it into vitamin D3. From there, vitamin D3 is transported to places in the body where it gets 'activated,' meaning it's ready for use by the body. Sun exposure accounts for about 90 per cent of the vitamin D in people who don't take supplements.

Even in Australia, those living in our major population centres are making very little of their own vitamin D3 through sun exposure during winter. It's thought that above latitudes of about 33 degrees, vitamin D3 synthesis in the skin is very low or absent during most of the winter. Sydney is at 34 degrees latitude and Melbourne at 38 degrees. There's some evidence, however, that vitamin D synthesis may be better at these latitudes south of the equator rather than north.

If someone with pale skin gets 'modest' sun exposure by lying outside in a swimsuit (meaning the skin isn't burnt, but lightly pink 24 hours later), they'll make 15 000–20 000 IU of vitamin D. Compare that with the amount of vitamin D in a glass of milk – about 100 IU. People who tan easily or have naturally dark skin have higher concentrations of melanin, the skin pigment, which blocks the sun's UVB rays. That means they need three to six times as much sun exposure to produce enough vitamin D.

Australians are great users of sunscreen – the stronger the better. Unfortunately, sunscreen with an SPF of 30 pretty effectively blocks UVB rays, reducing vitamin D production by 95 per cent.

Certain people are particularly at risk of vitamin D deficiency:

- those who spend a lot of time indoors
- those who wear clothes that prevent sunlight reaching the skin
- elderly people, especially those in residential care
- obese people
- those with naturally darker skin
- breastfed babies whose mothers have low vitamin D levels.

Can we get vitamin D from our diets?

As we've seen, we get most of our vitamin D from sun exposure. There are some dietary sources of vitamin D, but they won't fulfil your daily requirements.

Many people associate dairy with vitamin D, but there's not a huge amount of vitamin D in dairy products. There is more in products from grass-fed cows that spend time in the sun (generating their own vitamin D), and they need to be the full-fat varieties because vitamin D is fat-soluble. People on low-fat diets find it even harder to maintain adequate vitamin D levels.

The best food sources of vitamin D are:

- oily fish, such as salmon, trout, mackerel, sardines and tuna, and fish roe
- eggs
- mushrooms
- milk
- beef liver
- cod liver oil.

How can you tell if you're vitamin D deficient?

Your best bet is to get your vitamin D levels checked by your GP with a test called 25-hydroxy vitamin D [25(OH)D]. There's some controversy over the levels that should be considered adequate and those that equate to vitamin D deficiency. Most authorities agree that, at the end of winter, less than 30 nmol/L is severely deficient, and less than 50 nmol/L is deficient. But what is ideal?

> I would not be happy with anything less than 80 nmol/L.

Be careful when looking at online discussions of vitamin D – while the units used in Australia are nmol/L, in North America they use ng/ml, and 1 ng/ml = 2.5 nmol/L.

Status	Vitamin D level (nmol/L)
Severely deficient	<30
Deficient	<50
Sub-optimal	<80
Ideal	>80

How much vitamin D do we need?

This depends on a lot of things, but the short answer is that we need enough to keep our vitamin D levels in the optimal range (more than 80 nmol/L). The nutrient reference values (NRVs) for Australia and New Zealand are 200 IU (5 µg) a day for infants, children and adults below 50, 400 IU (10 µg) for those aged 50–70, and 600 IU (15 µg) for those over 70. The US Institute of Medicine's recommended daily allowance (RDA) for vitamin D is 600 IU. Many experts feel that these amounts are far too low, and some recommend as much as a 10-fold increase. I think 2000–4000 IU is a good amount for those who need it.

It doesn't take much sun exposure for the body to produce vitamin D. Even the most vocal supporters of unprotected sun exposure recommend no more than 10–15 minutes of exposure to arms, legs, abdomen and back, two or three times a week, followed by good sun protection.

If environmental conditions are optimal, a young adult man can create 10 000–20 000 IU (250–500 µg) of vitamin D daily from sunlight exposure. But the conditions aren't always optimal. Season, time of day, length of day, cloud cover, smog, skin melanin content and sunscreen are among the factors that affect UV radiation exposure and vitamin D synthesis. Having said that, even in high latitudes, we can form vitamin D from exposure to sunlight during the spring, summer and autumn months, and store it in the liver and fat for use in winter.

Complete cloud cover reduces UV by 50 per cent; shade (including that produced by severe pollution) reduces it by 60 per cent. UVB radiation doesn't penetrate glass, so exposure to sunshine indoors through a window doesn't produce vitamin D. Sunscreens with a sun protection factor (SPF) of 8 or more appear to block the UV rays needed to make vitamin D, although in practice people generally don't apply enough, cover all sun-exposed skin, or reapply sunscreen regularly, so their skin probably synthesises some vitamin D even when they're wearing sunscreen.

Some authorities recommend avoiding midday sun exposure when the sun emits more damaging rays. Those 'damaging' rays are, however, the very ones that your skin uses to make vitamin D. UVB rays are at their peak between roughly 10 a.m. and 2 p.m., so if you've been taking an early morning walk to get your vitamin D, you might want to reschedule (or spend some extra time outside in the middle of the day).

Should we take vitamin D supplements?

Again, there's a range of opinions on who needs a vitamin D supplement. If I was living in the northern hemisphere at a latitude where there was little winter sunshine, I would take supplements (or at least try and get away for a sunny holiday as often as I could). I don't think, though, that everyone living in Sydney or Melbourne, for instance, needs a supplement. Specific groups should probably use supplements wherever they live. These would include pregnant women, obese people and elderly people in residential care.

The key to whether you need a supplement is your vitamin D level. If your blood test shows you are deficient (less than 50 nmol/L) or even sub-optimal (less than 80 nmol/L), I would suggest taking a supplement until your levels are over 80 nmol/L. I would probably recommend

2000–4000 IU per day if you're deficient and you don't have the opportunity to get much vitamin D through sun exposure.

It's important to make sure that your supplement is in the form of D3 rather than D2, although most are D3 these days.

My approach to sun

I believe that getting adequate vitamin D, preferably through sun exposure, is very important. The first and most important advice regarding the sun is: *Don't get burnt.*

Avoiding sunburn is essential. The challenge then is to get adequate sun exposure without burning. I've always figured that there's a reason you have spring before summer – it gives you a chance to get your skin accustomed to sun and gradually increasing levels of intensity. So I take every opportunity to expose my skin to the sun for short periods – 10–15 minutes (or less if the sun is particularly fierce). If I need to stay in the sun longer than that, I apply sunscreen.

I get my vitamin D blood level checked each year, ideally at the end of winter. Fortunately, other than when I lived in the United Kingdom, I've never been in the deficient range. If I was, though, I would be very conscientious about getting sun exposure and, if that wasn't possible, I would take 2000–4000 IU of vitamin D3 a day.

POINTS TO REMEMBER
- To avoid skin cancers, we need to avoid getting sunburnt.
- We need mild to moderate exposure to the sun to produce sufficient vitamin D.
- Deficiency of vitamin D is associated with adverse health outcomes, so get your vitamin D levels checked and take a supplement if they're low.

Don't Smoke

Smoking is unhealthy. End of story.

It's hard to believe that well into the 21st century we're still talking about smoking. We've known for 50 years that smoking is harmful to our health, with clear links to lung cancer, emphysema and cardiovascular disease among others. And yet one in seven Australian men and women smoke. The numbers are coming down but very slowly.

	Smokers in 2015 (%)	Annual rate of change 1990–2015 (%)
Australian men	15.6	–1.9
Australian women	13.3	–2.1
UK men	19.9	–1.4
UK women	18.1	–1.4
US men	14.4	–2.0
US women	11.7	–2.2

Source: GBD 2015 Tobacco Collaborators, *Lancet*, 2017[1]

The latest figures show that in 2015, 6.4 million deaths were attributable to smoking worldwide – one in ten adults dies from tobacco-related illnesses. And for every death caused by a smoking-related disease, there are 20 more people living with at least one serious smoking-related illness.[1]

According to the 2014 US Surgeon General's Report (SGR), nearly 90 per cent of adult smokers started before the age of 18, and nearly all started by age 26. Of every three young smokers, only one will quit, and one of those remaining smokers will die from tobacco-related causes. Most of these young people never considered the long-term health consequences associated with tobacco use when they started smoking.[2]

Any kind of tobacco use has health risks. There are at least 250 chemicals in tobacco smoke that are toxic or cause cancer. A smoking habit of one to four cigarettes a day increases the chance of developing cardiovascular disease. Other known risks of nicotine addiction include

pneumonia, emphysema, chest infections, cataracts and other eye problems, and certain cancers, including those of the mouth, pharynx, larynx,
oesophagus, stomach, pancreas, cervix, kidney, ureter and bladder as well
as some forms of leukaemia.[3]

The risk of dying from lung cancer, or another kind of cancer, doubles
for smokers, and as many as 90 per cent of people diagnosed with lung
cancer are smokers. They're also more likely to suffer from gum disease,
insulin resistance, type 2 diabetes, infertility and pregnancy complications.
Smokers will also age prematurely and have yellow-stained, sallow skin.

> On average, non-smokers live about a decade longer than smokers

Nicotine is as addictive as cocaine or heroin. Just 1 milligram of the 10 milligrams in an average cigarette is enough to get you hooked. Most smokers
say they want to quit, but without help, more than 85 per cent of those
who try will start smoking again in about a week.[4]

Why is it so hard to quit tobacco?
Quitting tobacco completely or even cutting back causes symptoms of
nicotine withdrawal, which are both physical and mental. Physically, the
body reacts to the absence of nicotine. Mentally, giving up the habit means
a major behavioural change. And it can even be an emotional wrench.

Nicotine withdrawal isn't dangerous, but it can be uncomfortable. The
symptoms usually start within a few hours and reach their peak two or
three days later, when most of the nicotine and its by-products have left
the body. Withdrawal can last from a few days to several weeks, but they
improve with every day away from tobacco.

Nicotine withdrawal symptoms can include:

- dizziness (for a day or two after quitting)
- depression
- feelings of frustration, impatience and anger
- anxiety
- irritability
- insomnia, including trouble falling asleep and staying asleep, and having bad dreams or even nightmares

- difficulty concentrating
- restlessness or boredom
- headaches
- tiredness
- increased appetite
- slower heart rate
- constipation and gas
- cough, dry mouth, sore throat and runny nose
- chest tightness.

How to quit

If quitting smoking was easy, very few people would still be smoking. Quitting is HARD.

There are a number of different techniques used to help quit smoking:[5]

Cold turkey

Some people do manage to give up smoking there and then, without any medical aids and purely through willpower. Most people will feel extremely proud if they manage to give up using this method, especially as the success rate is only 5–10 per cent.

Tapering

This involves slowly reducing the amount of nicotine day by day or week by week. This means either gradually reducing the number of daily cigarettes, or changing to cigarettes with increasingly lower nicotine, or both. Tapering is usually done over a three- to four-week period. It's fairly effective, with success rates of around 35 per cent after a year.

Nicotine replacement

A variety of nicotine replacement therapy products are available over the counter or on prescription, and include gum, patches, nasal spray, inhalers, lozenges and tablets. They deliver nicotine in small and safe doses, giving just the right amount to help reduce cravings and withdrawal symptoms. Their levels of nicotine are much lower and less concentrated than the amount found in cigarettes and they don't contain any of the other damaging chemicals and toxins. They allow smokers to concentrate on breaking their behavioural addiction to smoking.

Breaking the behavioural addiction to smoking is just as important as dealing with the physical withdrawal symptoms. While trying to give up smoking, smokers should focus on avoiding situations and people that are most likely to induce the desire to smoke, and try to do another activity during their habitual smoking time.

Studies have shown that smokers who use nicotine replacement to help them stop smoking are twice as likely to stop for good. It's even more effective when used in conjunction with counselling, professional support and support at home.

Nicotine replacement should continue for the recommended 12 weeks but never more than six months. The idea is to start on a higher-dose product then gradually move to lower doses until you are ready to do without them completely. Someone using nicotine replacement must not smoke or they could end up with too much nicotine in their body and possibly nicotine overdose. They should also use only one type of nicotine replacement at a time.

Hypnotherapy

The idea is to hypnotise the smoker and make them believe they no longer need or want to smoke. The hypnotist helps the smoker relax body and mind, then 'reprograms' the smoker's subconscious mind, through suggestions and affirmations.

There's no convincing scientific evidence that hypnotherapy actually works, although some studies claim a 66 per cent success rate.

Acupuncture

In this traditional Chinese technique, very fine needles are inserted into the skin at various points thought to affect the smoking-related areas of the body. The needles are left for about half an hour and are then removed. Two tiny needles are then inserted into the earlobes and left there. When the smoker feels the urge to smoke, they touch the earlobe and their craving is meant to subside because the needle stimulates a part of the body that helps reduce the cravings. The treatment lasts for about two weeks, with several visits during the first week when the withdrawal symptoms are at their greatest. Studies show wildly varied success rates.

VAPING

The latest thing in tobacco use is e-cigarettes and other high-tech, fashionable electronic 'vaping' devices. They're touted as a safe way for smokers to give up, while also being decried as a gateway for kids to get hooked on nicotine.

What is an e-cigarette?

The electronic cigarette simulates smoking, and is promoted to be used where smoking isn't allowed. It's also marketed as a healthier option than smoking cigarettes because the user inhales only nicotine, and not the other harmful chemicals such as tar and carbon monoxide found in traditional cigarettes. Many say, however, that there hasn't been enough research into the long-term effects of inhaling nicotine vapour or the general safety of e-cigarettes.

E-cigarettes look and feel the same as regular cigarettes, but:

- apart from nicotine, don't contain the harmful substances, including tar, in regular cigarettes
- have no offensive odours
- might result in health benefits from smoking fewer regular cigarettes
- offer no second-hand smoke risks.

Are e-cigarettes safe?

The safety of e-cigarettes is a hot topic (sorry about that!). The general consensus is that while they're not 100 per cent safe (thanks to their nicotine), they're considerably safer than real cigarettes. While nicotine is the addictive component, most of the harm in regular cigarettes comes from the many other chemicals inhaled in the smoke.

An expert review from Public Health England in 2015 estimated that e-cigarettes were 95 per cent less harmful than the real thing. Although that figure is generally considered too high, most would agree that e-cigarettes are 80–85 per cent less harmful.[6]

Critics of e-cigarettes fear that kids will get hooked on nicotine through vaping and then move on to cigarettes for a bigger kick.

At this stage there's insufficient evidence to determine whether that's true.

Can e-cigarettes help you give up cigarettes?
E-cigarettes are marketed as a tool to help with quitting, but there's little evidence at the moment.

POINTS TO REMEMBER

- About 15 per cent of Australians smoke, despite knowing the dangers.
- Smoking is incredibly difficult to give up, although there are various techniques available to help smokers quit.
- E-cigarettes appear to be less harmful than regular cigarettes.

PART VII

Tackling the Modern Epidemics

At the start of the book I introduced the modern epidemics we're facing. Now that we've established where we've gone wrong and the lifestyle choices we should be making – based on the scientific evidence – I'll offer my advice on how we can tackle each of them specifically. The good news is, there's a lot that's in our control.

1. Obesity

The fatter we get, the greater the cost to our health and society.

As stated earlier, obesity is a huge problem in Australia. The rates of overweight and obesity are increasing yearly with two thirds of Australian men, half our women and at least a quarter of our children overweight or obese.

What causes obesity?

We have already discussed the fact that the previous two main theories of obesity have been largely been discredited: that eating fat makes you fat; and that if calories in are higher than calories out, you'll become overweight.

The Western world has been on a 40-year experiment to determine whether a low-fat diet can reduce levels of obesity and chronic disease. It is surely time to admit that this experiment has been a disastrous failure. It is time to change tack.

As the science shows, it is not eating fat that causes us to be fat – it is the sugar and processed foods that have led to a state of insulin resistance. So the key to losing weight is reversing that state of insulin resistance, and we start by cutting back on sugar. As we have seen sugar is everywhere – we are in the midst of a sugardemic.

The steps to losing weight

A low-carb, healthy-fat diet

- No sugar-sweetened drinks – soft drinks, fruit juices, fruit drinks, cordials, flavoured drinks (milks, coffees and teas)
- No starchy foods which are broken down to sugar – pasta, rice, potatoes
- No processed grains – white bread and bread products (muffins, crumpets, biscuits etc), breakfast cereals
- Avoid foods with hidden sugars – flavoured yoghurts, muesli bars, sauces and dressings

Instead, eat real food (grass-fed meat and dairy, fish, non-starchy vegetables, avocados, berries, nuts and olive oil).

By reducing your glucose and subsequent insulin load you will reverse your insulin resistance and lose weight as well as gaining other health benefits. The reason is simple. Avoiding or significantly reducing foods containing sugar, starches and carbohydrates, will decrease your body's demand for, and production of the hormone insulin. High insulin levels block your body's ability to access your stored excess body fat. With clever food choices you can normalise insulin levels and your body will be able to release energy from fat.

Exercise

Many people subscribe to the theory that it doesn't matter what we eat because we can run it off tomorrow. Unfortunately, that just doesn't work. Even if the discredited *calories in, calories out* theory was true, it would take huge amounts of exercise to run off a large meal or big drinking session. As I mentioned previously, you can't outrun a bad diet.[1] That is not to say that exercise is not important for health – as we have seen – is just that it is not a major factor in reducing obesity. We are actually doing more exercise than ever, but still our waistlines grow.[2]

Most people falsely believe that if they have a little (or a lot) of weight to lose, once they start exercising they'll lose weight. Unfortunately, if we start exercising and don't lose weight, we tend to want to give up. Even worse, we have overweight kids who are made to feel guilty for their weight and told to go outside, exercise and play sport.

It could be that the opposite is true – weight loss may encourage exercise. If you are overweight and lose weight then you're likely to be more inclined to exercise; the exercise will be easier as a result of your weight loss and therefore will be more enjoyable.

Other lifestyle choices

As previously mentioned, both sleep and stress play important roles in managing obesity. There is clear evidence that less sleep is associated with obesity, while many of us find it very difficult to lose weight when under high levels of stress.

POINTS TO REMEMBER

- Eating too much sugar and processed food is the main cause of obesity – not eating too much fat or too many calories.
- Obesity is associated with chronic diseases such as type 2 diabetes, heart disease, cancer, arthritis, asthma and many more.
- Exercise does not cancel out a bad diet; you need to change what you eat.

2. Type 2 Diabetes

Diabetes is a gateway disease to a range of devastating health conditions.

Earlier on I described the two types of diabetes, type 1 (T1D) and type 2 (T2D), and how type 1 diabetics produce virtually no insulin and require regular injections of insulin to survive, whereas type 2 diabetics produce too much insulin because their cells have become resistant to its effects.

Why is diabetes such a problem?

As I mentioned earlier, the reason diabetes is such a health concern is the high incidence of complications associated with being diabetic.

Diabetics have a higher incidence of:

Cardiovascular disease – angina, heart attacks, strokes
Nerve damage – numbness, loss of feeling
Foot damage – ulcers, amputations
Eye damage – blindness
Kidney disease – kidney failure
Dementia and Alzheimer's disease ('type 3 diabetes')
Skin infections – bacterial, fungal

The mechanism behind all these complications of diabetes has always been thought to be the effect of high blood glucose levels on organs, especially the small blood vessels (capillaries). Hence the prime objective of treatment was to reduce high blood sugar levels.

While this is undoubtedly true, it is not the whole picture. Insulin is toxic and the high insulin levels associated with insulin resistance and T2D can have a direct effect on organs.

How diabetes is diagnosed

A definitive diagnosis of diabetes is made on the basis of a series of standard blood tests:

- fasting blood glucose: greater than 7.0mmol/L
- haemoglobin A1c (HbA1c) – average blood sugar in the preceding 2–3-month period: greater than 6.5 per cent
- glucose tolerance – blood glucose results before and 2 hours after ingesting 75 grams of glucose
- serum insulin – not commonly performed: greater than 9 µIU/ml.

A number of signs can *suggest* diabetes or pre-diabetes, however, including:

- abdominal obesity – the apple shape
- symptoms such as fatigue, excessive thirst, headaches or recurrent infections
- high blood pressure
- darkening of the skin, usually found in body folds (called acanthosis nigricans)
- abnormal foot sensations
- deteriorating eyesight
- gum disease and tooth decay
- sleep apnoea and snoring
- cardiovascular disease
- infertility.

METABOLIC SYNDROME

You don't go from having a normal metabolism to T2D overnight – it is really the end stage of the process of insulin resistance.

An intermediate stage has been identified and labelled meta-bolic syndrome. It is thought that approximately a quarter to a third of the adult population suffer from this syndrome.

Metabolic syndrome is a clustering of at least three of these five medical conditions:

- Abdominal (central) obesity: waist circumference ≥102 cm (males), ≥88 cm (females)
- Elevated blood pressure: >130 systolic or > 85 diastolic
- Elevated fasting blood glucose: >5.5mmol/L
- High serum triglycerides: >1.7mmol/L

> - Low high-density lipoprotein (HDL) levels: <1.0 mmol/L in men, <1.3 mmol/L in women
>
> In 1988, in his Banting lecture, Gerald M. Reaven named this constellation of abnormalities Syndrome X and proposed insulin resistance as the underlying factor. More recently the name was changed to Metabolic Syndrome and often abbreviated to MetSy. Reaven did not include abdominal obesity, which has since been added.

An incurable progressive disease?

Right through medical school and ever since, I have been taught that diabetes is a progressive disease – you can't prevent it and you can't reverse it. But that's not true – not for T2D, at least.

Another way of describing diabetes is to call it a disease of *carbohydrate intolerance*. It seems to me that if you have a condition where the underlying problem is an inability to metabolise carbohydrates, then the obvious treatment is to restrict your intake of carbohydrates. This *was* the preferred treatment of T2D, and as an adjunct to insulin injections for T1D, until the 1970s, when the Western world became obsessed with fat.

Fat, not carbohydrate, was deemed to be the health villain, and the priority became reducing dietary fat intake. Given that the protein levels in most diets stays the same, at 15–20 per cent of calories, if you want to reduce fat you have to replace it with carbohydrates, and that's what happened after the dietary guidelines were introduced in the early 1980s.

Ever since, the official dietary recommendations for diabetics have been the same as for the general population: low fat, high carbohydrates. We went from a carb/protein/fat ratio of something like 30/20/50 in the past to 65/20/15 in recent years. At the same time, the types of fat recommended changed from healthy animal-derived saturated fat to artificial polyunsaturated fats in the form of vegetable oils.

People with T2D have been encouraged to continue with this high-carbohydrate diet, which guarantees that their diabetes will persist and probably get worse. The medical profession's solution is then drugs. A whole range of drugs have been developed to treat type 2 diabetes, most commonly metformin tablets and insulin injections. These drugs have some success in lowering blood-glucose levels, but they actually worsen long-term outcomes because they don't address the primary problem – the high levels of insulin in the blood, known as hyperinsulinemia.

When you think about it, injecting insulin into someone with T2D who already has high insulin levels doesn't make a lot of sense. What is the solution to this dilemma?

A low-carbohydrate diet

There is one way of keeping both blood glucose and insulin levels low in people with T1D or T2D or anyone else for that matter: a low carbohydrate intake. This will allow the T1D sufferer to reduce their insulin dose while maintaining good blood glucose level (similarly in the T2Ds who are on insulin). Those with T2D not on insulin will benefit from reduced insulin resistance and gain the benefits of lower blood insulin levels.

As I have mentioned previously, the amount of carbs you should eat depends on your degree of insulin resistance. If you are relatively insulin sensitive, then you can eat a moderate amount of carbs, but if you are highly insulin resistant then you should severely limit your carb intake. By the time you have developed T2D, you are almost certainly highly insulin resistant, so you need to severely limit your carb intake.

When you are diagnosed with T2D, you should immediately go on a strict low-carb diet. Ideally you should limit your carb intake to 20–30 grams per day, which in reality is pretty much no carbs other than those found in green vegetables and some nuts. This is the ketogenic diet described earlier (page 179). By adjusting your carb intake, the goal is to get your blood insulin and glucose levels under control (to normal levels). Then you can continue to adjust your carb intake and find the level that is appropriate for you and your body's level of insulin resistance. The ultimate goal is to eliminate your insulin resistance.

Don't try this on your own. Reducing your carb intake will significantly lower your insulin and glucose levels and you may need to reduce or even cease your medication. You should have your blood sugar levels monitored regularly in the early stages of this process. Take your doctor on your journey. If he or she is reluctant to come on board, give them a copy of this book!

A review of the medical research into the use of low-carb diets in type 2 diabetics was published in 2015 and stated that this form of diet 'reliably reduces blood glucose levels' while reducing or eliminating the need for medication.[1] More recently, the Virta Group in the US have shown that an online programme with intensive nutrition and behavioural counselling, digital coaching and physician-guided medication management can be successful in reversing type 2 diabetes. More than 75 per cent of those on the low-carb diet had reduced their HbA1c measurement below the diabetes threshold as well as losing weight and reducing their medications.[2]

So really the recommended diet is the same for both T1D and T2D sufferers. In both cases adopting this diet will result in better blood glucose control, reduced medications (tablets or insulin) and reduction in the complications of diabetes. A no-brainer – and yet doctors and dietitians still tell their diabetic patients to eat lots of carbs. Unbelievable!

Other lifestyle choices

Lifestyle modification is the key to successfully managing type 2 diabetes and this involves primarily diet (which I've already discussed), but also improvements in exercise levels, sleep and stress reduction.

POINTS TO REMEMBER

- Diabetes is a disease of carbohydrate intolerance.
- Type 1 diabetes requires regular insulin injections, whereas type 2 diabetics produce too much insulin because their cells have become resistant to its effects.
- Type 2 diabetes is actually reversible, and both types benefit from a low-carb healthy-fat diet – consult your doctor about significantly reducing your carbohydrate intake, such as trying a ketogenic diet.

---

3. Fatty Liver

Many of us have a fatty liver and we don't even know it.

I previously drew your attention to the hidden epidemic of Non-Alcoholic Fatty Liver Disease (NAFLD) or fatty liver. Fatty liver is thought to be present in approximately one third of all adults in the Western world and yet most people are blissfully unaware of their problem.

Fatty liver is associated with a number of our major health issues including insulin resistance, diabetes and cardiovascular disease. It is thought to be a step on the way to developing T2D. As world-renowned Professor Roy Taylor, Professor of Medicine and Metabolism at Newcastle University, said: 'before diagnosis of Type 2 diabetes, there is a long silent scream from the liver'.

Fatty liver is also associated with the progressive liver disease known as non-alcoholic steatohepatitis (NASH) and with an increased incidence of liver cancer. It is predicted to lead to a massive increase in the number of liver transplants performed.

What causes fatty liver?

Fatty liver (foie gras) in ducks and geese is caused by overfeeding with sugars and starches and it is the same in humans. It seems that fructose is the major culprit.[1] Fructose constitutes 50 per cent of table sugar and a similar proportion in the widely used sugar substitute high fructose corn syrup (HFCS), and occurs naturally in fruit and fruit juice.

I have described previously the process by which glucose is produced from dietary carbohydrates and absorbed into the bloodstream, causing the pancreas to release insulin. The insulin then helps distribute the glucose to all the body's cells, where it is used for energy or stored as glycogen, with excess glucose being converted to fat.

Fructose, unlike glucose, is metabolised only in the liver and with no process by which it can be stored, is turned into fat through a process known as lipogenesis. Triglycerides are produced which accumulate as fat in both the liver and around the viscera (internal) organs, causing the apple shape belly described below. Fatty liver leads to insulin resistance and ultimately to type 2 diabetes.

Sugar is clearly the main culprit, with the dual adverse effects of its glucose (through hyperinsulinemia) and fructose (through fatty liver) leading to obesity and type 2 diabetes.

How do I know if I have fatty liver?

Fatty liver does not create any particular symptoms until it's well advanced. It is, however, associated with fat around the abdomen – the so-called apple shape (as opposed to the pear shape, where most of the fat is around the buttocks and thighs). A 'sugar belly', where your waist is larger than your hips, could indicate that you have a fatty liver. Fatty liver is often associated with high blood triglyceride levels, so if a blood test has shown this, you should request that your GP order a liver function test.

Liver function tests measure a number of enzymes in the blood (with helpful designations like ALT and GGT) that are associated with liver function. These are high in people with fatty liver. You may remember from earlier that my own blood tests had indicated impaired liver function over a ten-year period. Both my GGT and ALT were well above the normal values. The report always came back saying 'abnormal liver function consistent with fatty liver'. I'm embarrassed to say that I completely ignored those results and carried on as before. I didn't really understand what a fatty liver was; I figured I wasn't 'fat' and as I was eating a low-fat diet, I'd be fine.

Silly me. I changed my eating habits to reduce sugar, vegetable oils and starches, and replaced processed foods with real food. Three months later my blood results were perfectly normal, for instance my ALT which ideally should be below 40 came down from 65 to 25, and my GTT which should be less than 50 reduced from 56 to 21. Amazing! And what drug did I take to achieve this? A drug called FOOD!

Dealing with fatty liver

Fatty liver should not be ignored. It is a sign that insulin resistance is developing and is a precursor to type 2 diabetes. Fortunately it is reversible by avoiding sugar and processed foods.

Since sugar is the primary cause of fatty liver, reducing your intake of sugar is the key to both preventing and treating fatty liver. My own experience shows fatty liver can be reversed in as little time as three months by eating a diet low in sugar and processed foods. Don't forget: sugar is present in the majority of processed foods, so stick to real food.

Fruit is a major source of fructose, so it's important to limit your fruit intake if you have fatty liver. Restricting yourself to a couple of pieces of fruit a day is probably ideal, and the best fruits to eat are berries, which are relatively low in sugars. Generally speaking, the sweeter a fruit tastes, the higher its sugar content, so avoid the really sweet fruits such as mangoes and grapes. Small amounts of whole fruits such as an apple are absorbed slowly and don't produce a rapid intake of fructose for the liver to deal with. The main problem is the fructose in fruit juice and soft drinks.

POINTS TO REMEMBER
- Fatty liver is a common condition affecting as many as one third of adults.
- Fatty liver is caused by an excess intake of sugar and processed foods.
- Fatty liver can be reversed by following a low-sugar, real-food lifestyle.

---

4. Tooth Decay

Sugar destroys teeth.

As mentioned previously, one in three Australian children aged 5–6 years have tooth decay in their deciduous (baby) teeth, and two in five children aged 10–12 years have tooth decay in their permanent (adult) teeth. Around 90 per cent of adults have experienced tooth decay in their lifetime.

Dental caries is caused by the action of acids on the enamel surface. The acid is produced when bacteria present in the dental biofilm (plaque) on the tooth surface break down fermentable carbohydrates such as sugar (sucrose). The acid produced leads to a loss of calcium and phosphate from the enamel – this process is called demineralisation.

Saliva acts to dilute and neutralise the acid which causes demineralisation and is an important natural defence against caries. Aside from buffering plaque acids and halting the demineralisation of enamel, saliva provides a reservoir of minerals adjacent to the enamel from which it can remineralise and 'heal' once the acids have been neutralised.

The enamel demineralises and remineralises many times during the course of a day. It is when this balance is upset and demineralisation exceeds remineralisation that caries progresses. When demineralisation occurs frequently and exceeds remineralisation over many months, there is a breakdown of the enamel surface leading to a cavity.

The role of sugar in tooth decay in absolutely clear. There is a mountain of evidence that demonstrates that both the amount and frequency of sugar consumption is strongly associated with tooth decay.[1] Sugar-sweetened soft drinks have been shown to increase the risk of tooth decay, and more than 50 per cent of Australian children drink at least one sugar-sweetened drink a day.[2]

Tackling tooth decay

Given the overwhelming evidence that frequent consumption of sugars is associated with tooth decay, the dietary advice should be aimed at reducing sugar intake and its frequency. Studies have shown that even when populations have adequate exposure to fluoride, sugar consumption remains a moderate risk factor for tooth decay.[3]

We need to be aware of the foods and drinks that contain 'free sugars' – sugars that have been added to food plus those naturally present in honey, fruit juices and syrup – and reduce how often we eat them, particularly between meals. Eating sugar between meals increases the periods when the plaque becomes too acidic and demineralisation begins. Bear in mind, too, that though diet and sugar-free soft drinks have a reduced sugar content, they're still highly acidic and can erode tooth enamel.[4]

It's critical to brush and floss our teeth at least twice a day with a fluoridated toothpaste to reduce the number of plaque bacteria, and to teach our children to do the same. It's also vital to teach our children well by ensuring their diet is low in sugars and fermentable carbohydrates.

Gum disease

There also appears to be a relationship between poor diet and gum disease, which is probably not surprising, given gum disease is due to inflammation – and we have already discussed the impact of diet on inflammation earlier in this book. A recent German study showed that a diet low in carbohydrates but rich in omega-3 fatty acids, vitamins C and D, antioxidants and fibre significantly reduced gum inflammation.[5]

POINTS TO REMEMBER
- Tooth cavities are due to demineralisation of the tooth enamel as a result of excess acid production.
- Frequent consumption of sugars is associated with tooth decay.
- Reducing both the amount and frequency of sugar consumption is essential to prevent tooth decay.

5. Cardiovascular Disease

We need to rethink our approach to our leading cause of death.

While the mortality from cardiovascular disease (CVD) has decreased slightly over the past couple of decades, it is still a massive problem in our society and, with cancer, one of the two leading causes of death. The reduction in mortality is probably largely due to a combination of reduced smoking and better emergency care of those who have heart attacks. There is even some recent evidence that the incidence of CVD might be starting to increase again, probably due to the increasing incidence of obesity and diabetes.[1]

What causes cardiovascular disease?

The truth is we don't actually know. We're starting to get an idea, however, and it's probably quite different from what we've thought for the past few decades.

As I explained early on in the book, for the past 50 years we've been working on the assumptions of the diet–heart theory first proposed by US physiologist Ancel Keys. The research this theory was based on was, however, of dubious quality. The diet–heart theory claims that cholesterol is the main cause of atherosclerosis, and that by reducing our intake of dietary cholesterol and saturated fat, we can significantly reduce our chance of developing CVD.

But that hasn't proven to be the case. Since the dietary guidelines have kept people from eating too much cholesterol or saturated fat, the CVD figures have hardly changed, and we've seen a steady increase in obesity, type 2 diabetes and other chronic diseases. Even the use of statin medications, which markedly reduce blood-cholesterol readings, have made hardly any difference.

As I have stated elsewhere in this book, when prominent researcher Zoë Harcombe recently went back and looked at the scientific evidence available at the time the diet–heart hypothesis became popular, she was unable to find any evidence at all. Nor has there been significant evidence in the 50 years since.

I am certainly not suggesting that cholesterol does not play a role in the development of atherosclerosis, but it is not as simple as high blood cholesterol levels leading to atherosclerosis. There are many people with low cholesterol who have heart attacks and many with high levels who do not.

The role of LDL particles

We previously thought that high levels of cholesterol and particularly high levels of the LDL ('bad' cholesterol) particles that transport cholesterol and triglycerides around the blood led to cholesterol plaque formation. The plaque both narrowed the lumen of the artery and was also prone to thrombus formation (blood clots) and rupture, which caused heart attacks and strokes.

Now it seems it's not the total number of LDL particles that's important, but how many of those particles are oxidised (*oxLDL*). Normal LDL particles keep moving around in the bloodstream, while oxidised particles finish up sticking to the artery walls and starting off the atherosclerosis process.

The LDL particle can be oxidised for a variety of reasons. One is excess intake of omega-6 fats, particularly from hydrogenated vegetable oils. LDL can also become oxidised if it stays in the blood too long, and if it's exposed to excessive glucose and fructose levels after meals, or to smoking and other stressors.

When LDL particles are oxidised, they cause an inflammatory reaction in the lining of the arteries where white blood cells attempt to engulf the oxidised LDL and the cholesterol it's carrying. It's this inflammatory process that leads to plaque formation. Initially the plaque may be relatively stable and harmless, but if the numbers of damaged LDL particles continue to be high, the plaque can become vulnerable to rupture, leading to heart attacks and strokes.

Avoiding smoking, reducing intake of omega-6 fats by avoiding hydrogenated vegetable oils, and reducing sugar intake are three simple ways that oxidation of LDL and inflammation can be reduced. The high-carbohydrate, low-fat diet, recommended for the past 40 years, is more likely to produce smaller LDL particles, which are more susceptible to oxidisation than the larger, fluffier particles that result when carbo-hydrate intake is reduced. The LDL particles can also be damaged by a process called glycation, where a sugar molecule attaches to the LDL, making it more vulnerable to oxidation.

Our old friend insulin resistance is associated with many of the factors that contribute to the development of atherosclerosis, such as low HDL and high levels of triglyceride-rich particles. Increased numbers of small LDL particles susceptible to oxidisation are also common in people with insulin resistance.

The HDL ('good' cholesterol) particles transport some of the choles-terol from the damaged LDL particles back to the liver for disposal as bile salts and acids. This is known as reverse cholesterol transport.

Phew. That was complicated. So what does it all mean for the prevention of heart attacks?

Treating cardiovascular disease

From what we learnt above about the causes of CVD, it makes sense that anything that could:

- reduce the number of small LDL particles
- increase the number of protective HDL particles, and
- reduce the oxidisation and glycation of LDL

might help reduce the incidence of CVD.

Low-carbohydrate diets provide greater improvements in parameters associated with insulin resistance, such as HDL cholesterol, LDL parti-cle size and particle number. Moreover, low-carbohydrate diets provide greater reductions in inflammatory markers than low-fat diets.

The best way to avoid heart disease is to avoid insulin resistance with a low-sugar, nutrient-dense, real-food lifestyle. And yet most doctors will recommend a high-carb low-fat diet and reach for the prescription pad.

Exercise has been shown to be beneficial for those with CVD. Moderate to high levels of fitness have been shown to be associated with reduced mortality from cardiovascular disease and can reduce the risks associated with a high TG/HDL ratio.[2]

STATINS

Statins are a class of drugs prescribed to lower cholesterol levels with the aim of reducing CVD risk. The statins available in Australia are atorvastatin (Lipitor), fluvastatin (Lescol), pravastatin (Pravachol), rosuvastatin (Crestor) and simvastatin (Zocor). Statins are the most successful drugs in history, with annual sales of $33 billion worldwide. More than 20 million prescriptions are written in Australia each year. There is considerable debate in medical circles about the extent to which statins should be prescribed.

Originally statins were only recommended for those with established CVD, such as those who'd already had a heart attack or angina. The scientific evidence overall supports the use of statins in these people, although this may be because they help reduce inflammation rather than lowering cholesterol. There is also evidence that for people without evidence of established CVD yet who are at high risk of CVD, such as those with high blood pressure or a strong family history of CVD, preventative treatment with statins reduces the risk of all-cause death, heart attack, stroke and need for heart surgery with no evidence of any serious harm.[3]

While there is clearly benefit from the use of statins in those with established CVD and those at high risk, the use of statins in those with elevated cholesterol but otherwise at low risk of CVD is being increasingly questioned. Elevated total cholesterol levels are no longer thought to be a good indicator of risk for CVD, and even the role of elevated LDL-cholesterol is being debated.

The results of trials in older (>65) people suggest that there is no advantage to taking statins in this group and, in fact, in the elderly the lower the cholesterol, the more likely they are to die.[4]

There is also considerable disagreement about the frequency and seriousness of the side effects of statins. These include muscle aches, weakness, fatigue, digestive problems, cognitive dysfunction including short-term memory loss, erectile dysfunction, sleep disorders, cataracts and type 2 diabetes.

So unless you have established heart disease, or are at high risk

> of CVD, you don't necessarily need to take a statin. You'd be much better off improving your diet by reducing your intake of sugar, vegetable oils and processed foods, and focusing on eating nutrient-dense real food, exercising regularly, not smoking, reducing stress, improving sleep and getting out into the sun more often.

Are you at risk of cardiovascular disease?

Traditionally, doctors have calculated CVD risk by comparing a number of markers, such as total cholesterol and LDL levels, and with scales such as the Framingham Risk Score. Unfortunately, these markers and scores are all dependent on total cholesterol levels.

There are two very good measures of CVD risk. The first is your triglyceride to HDL ratio, which you can calculate yourself from your standard fasting cholesterol and triglyceride test. Simply divide your trig level by your HDL level (or use an online calculator).[5] This ratio is also a good indicator of insulin resistance, which we know is a key underlying factor in the development of CVD.[6] A ratio of less than 1.5 means you're at low risk of CVD. In fact, one study found that the people in the top 25 per cent for triglyceride to HDL ratio had a 16 times higher risk of heart disease than those in the bottom 25 per cent.[7]

The other, more sophisticated (and expensive) test is the coronary artery calcium (CAC) score. This is determined with a CT scan and measures the amount of calcium plaques in the walls of the arteries around the heart. There's good correlation between CAC score and CVD risk.[8] A CAC score of zero means a very low risk of heart attack. Once the CAC score goes above 10, the risk starts to increase. Once your CAC score is over 1000, your risk of a heart attack is quite high. Increasing CAC scores over time are also a risk.

The CAC test costs about $150–200 and currently has no Medicare rebate, but it's a couple of hundred bucks well spent. A zero or low score is very reassuring.

So, it appears that the best way to avoid heart disease is to avoid insulin resistance. And we know the best way to do that is with a low-sugar, nutrient-dense, real food lifestyle. Easy!

POINTS TO REMEMBER

- The cause of CVD is complex but involves excessive sugar and processed foods, insulin resistance and inflammation.
- The triglyceride to HDL ratio and CAC score are the two best predictors of CVD.
- The best way to avoid CVD is with a low-sugar, nutrient-dense, real-food lifestyle. Statins are only of use to people with established CVD or those at high risk of CVD.

6. Chronic Diseases

Poor diet is implicated in a wide range of debilitating conditions.

I have already told you about the link between what we eat and the modern epidemics of obesity, T2D, fatty liver, dental caries and cardiovascular disease. For all these conditions, there is good evidence of the role that poor nutrition, especially high intakes of sugar, vegetable oils and processed foods, has in their development.

But there is another group of chronic diseases for which evidence is starting to emerge about their link with what we eat.

Unfortunately, nutrition research is not 'sexy' and struggles to attract funding given that the major funders of medical research are the pharmaceutical companies, who have no interest in showing that good nutrition might work better than drugs for certain diseases. For most of these conditions, there is not sufficient evidence as yet to categorically state that there is a link between these chronic diseases and what we eat – but there is enough out there even now to be highly suspicious. Hopefully over the next few years, more and more evidence will emerge.

Dementia and Alzheimer's

Dementia is not one specific disease but rather a collection of symptoms caused by different disorders of which Alzheimer's disease is the most common.

Alzheimer's disease is rapidly increasing in prevalence. It is a condition in which abnormal proteins aggregate to form plaques and tangles in the brain, which then progressively damage the brain and lead to severe cognitive decline. It slowly and progressively robs people of their ability to think, move, communicate and live everyday life. It has a devastating effect both on the individual sufferer and their extended family.

There is a lot of interest in the link between nutrition and dementia and Alzheimer's. In fact, Alzheimer's disease has been described as 'type 3 diabetes', such is the strength of the suspected link to type 2 diabetes.[1]

We know that diabetes patients are more likely to develop Alzheimer's disease. Researchers are suggesting that the brain may develop insulin resistance, leading to high levels of glucose that then attaches to certain proteins, damaging the brain and impairing insulin signalling.[2]

A group of British researchers recently suggested that there was a 'tipping point', beyond which glucose levels start to impair the action of a protein that would normally counteract the build-up of abnormal proteins that occurs in the early stages of Alzheimer's.[3]

Another study showed that the more sugary drinks consumed, the lower the total brain volume and the lower the scores on memory tests. Compared with those who drank no sugary drinks, those who drank one or two a day had a reduced brain volume equivalent to 1.6 years of normal ageing, and lower memory scores equivalent to 5.8 years of ageing. Those who drank more than two sugary drinks a day had decreased brain volume equivalent to two years of normal ageing and lower memory scores equivalent to 11 years of ageing.[4] Brain shrinkage is associated with an increased risk of Alzheimer's disease.

As high blood glucose levels in the brain are a factor in the development of Alzheimer's, it makes sense to reduce them. Contrary to what many believe, the brain needs very little glucose to survive. When required, the body can produce more than enough glucose from protein and fat by a process known as gluconeogenesis, so there's no need for much dietary glucose. The brain has an alternative fuel – ketones – on which it can function just as well as with glucose. The best way to switch the brain's fuel from glucose to ketones is to start a ketogenic diet (see page 179).

A small study conducted at the University of Kansas that looked at the effect of a ketogenic diet on people with Alzheimer's disease showed impressive improvements on the Alzheimer's cognition scale.[5] Another study looked at the use of a very low-carbohydrate diet in those with mild cognitive impairment, thought to be a precursor to Alzheimer's disease, and found improved memory performance.[6]

A possible approach for Alzheimer's and dementia

If someone near and dear to me started developing the first signs of Alzheimer's, I'd strongly urge them to commence a strict ketogenic diet, while ensuring regular exercise, adequate sleep and plenty of sun. While there's no guarantee this intervention would reverse or even halt the progression of the disease, there's enough evidence to convince me it's worth a try. Better still, adopt a low-sugar, low-vegetable-oil eating habit focusing on real foods throughout your life, and you might be able to prevent or delay the onset of Alzheimer's.

Cancer

Now before anybody goes off and claims that crazy Brukner bloke is saying you can cure cancer with diet, let me say that there is no evidence that diet can 'cure cancer', but there is some interesting evidence coming to light that there may be a role for diet as an adjunct to the more traditional cancer treatments.

It has been known for almost a century that cancer cells rely heavily on glucose as a fuel. This was first described by the Nobel prize winner Otto Warburg and colleagues in 1923 and is known as the Warburg effect.[7] In a normal cell, one glucose molecule will produce 38 ATP molecules (the units of energy), whereas in a cancer cell a glucose molecule will only produce two ATPs. As a result, massive amounts of glucose are needed to keep up with the energy demands of cancer cells.

When energy metabolism shifts to burning fat (in the form of ketones) rather than glucose, the cancer cells, which can't utilise ketones, are starved while our healthy cells can continue as normal.[8] There's some evidence from animal studies of a dramatic impairment of cancer growth when cells are deprived of glucose as a fuel using a strict ketogenic diet.[9] A few case reports and pre-clinical studies have yielded promising results in cancer patients as well.[10] Several registered clinical trials are currently investigating the case for a ketogenic diet as a supportive (not alternative) therapy with traditional cancer treatments.

Cancer is characterised by chronic inflammation and associated with insulin resistance. The beneficial effects of calorie restriction and fasting on cancer risk and progression are well established.[11] Carbohydrate restriction thus opens the possibility of targeting the same underlying mechanisms without the side effects of hunger and weight loss.

A possible approach for cancer

If I were diagnosed with cancer, I would adopt a dual approach. I'd get the best advice possible from an oncologist and follow their recommendations for any combination of surgery, radiation and chemotherapy. In addition, I'd immediately commence a two- to three-day fast and then adopt a strict ketogenic diet to deprive the cancer cells of the glucose they need for growth, while at the same time providing my healthy cells with ketones as a fuel source. I'd also exercise as regularly as possible, ensure I got plenty of good-quality sleep, try to reduce my stress levels, and get plenty of sunshine.

Neurological diseases

While there's a long history of the use of diet in the management of epilepsy, more recently other neurological diseases have been studied.

Epilepsy

Epilepsy is a chronic neurological disorder associated with a disruption in the normal electrical activity in the brain. The main symptom is repeated seizures, which can range from brief lapses to severe and prolonged convulsions. It's a variable condition that can differ in its impact from person to person. There are, for example, more than 40 different types of seizure that people with epilepsy can experience. Epilepsy, which affects 50 million people worldwide, is classed as one of the most common neurological diseases and can occur at any age. The cause of epilepsy is usually unknown, but in about 30 per cent of cases it occurs as a result of brain damage, head trauma, stroke, tumour or infection.

Epilepsy is treated in both children and adults with drugs known as anti-epileptic medications (AEDs). Epilepsy is well controlled in about 70 per cent of those on these medications. Some people with epilepsy, however, suffer from intractable seizures.

Since the 1920s, the treatment in this case has been with a ketogenic diet. Before the advent of AEDs, a ketogenic diet was the primary treatment for epilepsy, but after these medications appeared, the diet was ignored for many years. Recently, however, there has been renewed interest in treatment with a ketogenic diet for the 30 per cent or so of epileptics who are not well controlled with medication. Research seems to indicate that about

50 per cent of those with intractable epilepsy achieve good control when treated with a ketogenic diet.[12]

The exact link between the ketones produced with a ketogenic diet and the anticonvulsant effect isn't fully understood, but it's believed that the ketones both provide this effect while also reducing neuronal excitability in the brain. Another hypothesis is that ketones work by affecting the main excitatory and inhibitory neurotransmitters, GABA and glutamate.[13]

The Charlie Foundation for Ketogenic Therapies was founded in 1994 to provide information about diet therapies for people with epilepsy, other neurological disorders and select cancers. In 1993, 11-month-old Charlie Abrahams developed difficult-to-control epilepsy, with multiple daily seizures and medications. In desperation, his parents turned to a ketogenic diet and it worked. Within a month, Charlie was seizure- and drug-free. After five years on the diet he switched to eating whatever he wants and has never had another seizure.[14]

Other neurological diseases

In other neurological conditions, such as Parkinson's disease, multiple sclerosis (MS), amyotrophic lateral sclerosis (ALS), motor neurone disease (MND), autism and migraines, there is much anecdotal but very limited scientific evidence linking improvements with dietary interventions such as the ketogenic diet.

One interesting case is that of Dr Terry Wahls, a physician and clinical professor of medicine at the University of Iowa's Carver College of Medicine in Iowa City. In 2000, Terry was diagnosed with MS and three years later was confined to a wheelchair. In late 2007 she commenced a diet of 'greens, sulfur-rich vegetables, deeply colored vegetables and berries, grass-fed meat, wild fish, organ meat, and seaweed'. Nine months later she completed a 29-kilometre bike ride.[15]

Mental illness

There's been considerable interest in the past few years in possible links between nutrition and mental illness. Some psychiatrists are now advocating using nutrition as an adjunct to the more traditional treatments.

Recently, Australian researchers at Deakin University published the results of a randomised controlled trial that tested whether improving diet quality could treat clinical depression. The people in the trial were divided into two groups. In addition to medication the first group received dietary information and advice on improving the quality of their current diet, with a focus on increasing intake of fresh fruit and vegetables, whole grains, legumes, healthy meats, olive oil and nuts, while cutting down on unhealthy foods, such as confectionery, refined cereals, fried foods, fast food, processed meats and sugary drinks.

This group experienced a much greater reduction in their depressive symptoms over a three-month period than the second group, which received social support, also known to be helpful for people with depression. At the end of the trial, a third of those in the dietary support group were considered to be in remission for major depression, compared to 8 per cent of those in the social support group.[16]

In a separate study, the same Deakin University researchers showed an association between low intake of red meat in women and a diagnosed depressive or anxiety disorder. On the other hand, excessive intake of red meat was also associated with increased depression and anxiety.[17]

I'd certainly advise anyone with a mental illness to try a strict real-food, low-processed-food diet, along with regular exercise, as an adjunct to their other treatment.

Arthritis

Let me start by telling you a story.

One of my patients, an international cricketer, had suffered from knee pain for a couple of years. He was having difficulty playing and was on a reduced training load. He'd also put on some weight. Despite seeing multiple specialists and having numerous investigations including a knee arthroscopy, no one could work out what was wrong with him. Eventually a rheumatologist diagnosed him with 'sero-negative arthritis', a form of arthritis similar to rheumatoid arthritis.

The specialist started the cricketer on some powerful drugs, which led to a slight improvement in symptoms, then changed him to etanercept, an even more powerful (and expensive) drug. When I first met him, the player was injecting himself with etanercept every fortnight. He told me that after ten days his knee would start to hurt and he knew it was time for his next injection.

He approached me about trying a low-carb healthy-fat diet, primarily to try to lose some of the weight he'd put on. He embraced the diet enthusiastically and was very strict with his reduced carb intake. Three weeks later he came to me a bit sheepishly and admitted that he'd forgotten to inject his etanercept the previous week because he hadn't had any knee pain. He wanted to know whether he should inject it anyway. I suggested he wait to see if he developed any pain.

One year later he was still pain-free and off all medication. Apart from saving the $15000 a year the drug was costing, he'd dropped a few kilograms and was now able to complete full training sessions. I must admit even I was amazed at the dramatic improvement.

Overweight or obese patients with arthritis of the hip, knee or ankle are usually advised to try to lose weight in order to reduce the load on the joint. When placed on a low-carb healthy-fat diet they'll usually lose some weight and experience reduction in their joint pain. I would suggest, however, that this isn't due to the weight loss itself, but rather to the effect of reduced sugar intake on the level of inflammation.

Autoimmune diseases

Autoimmune diseases occur when inflammation causes the body to attack its own tissues. Autoimmune diseases can affect single organs (local autoimmune disease), or a number of organs or tissues (systemic autoimmune disease).

Local autoimmune diseases include conditions affecting the gut (coeliac and Crohn's disease, ulcerative colitis), thyroid (Graves' and Hashimoto's disease), liver (autoimmune hepatitis, primary biliary cirrhosis), adrenal gland (Addison's disease), pancreas (type 1 diabetes) and nervous system (Guillain-Barré syndrome, multiple sclerosis). Systemic autoimmune diseases include rheumatoid arthritis, scleroderma, Sjögren's syndrome, fibromyalgia and lupus.

It's been suggested that these autoimmune diseases are linked with leaky gut syndrome (see page 62). Anyone with these diseases should do everything they can to limit inflammation – a healthy diet, improved sleep, stress reduction and regular exercise.

Other diseases

Other disorders where there is substantial anecdotal, but minimal scientific, evidence of improvement with diets such as the ketogenic, low-carb or Paleo diets include:

- Fibromyalgia
- Chronic fatigue syndrome
- Allergies
- Asthma
- Tendinopathy
- GERD (gastroesophageal reflux disease)

POINTS TO REMEMBER
- There is some evidence that diseases such as dementia, epilepsy, cancer and autoimmune diseases may be linked to poor diet.
- Childhood epilepsy has been treated effectively with a ketogenic diet for many years.
- As cancer cells rely on glucose for fuel, it has been suggested that depriving those cells of glucose with a low-sugar diet may be an effective adjunct to traditional cancer treatments.

Conclusion

I hope by now you've realised that many of the things I've written about are interrelated. Here are key the messages that I really want you to take away with you to lead a happier, healthier life.

The Final Challenge

To finish, I set myself one final challenge: to sum up the keys to a healthy lifestyle in just two pages. If I had to summarise this book in one paragraph, this would be it:

> Adopting a way of eating that revolves around low sugar, minimal processed foods and avoidance of vegetable oils, and replacing them with plenty of nutrient-dense real foods, will have positive effects on insulin resistance, your lipid profile, inflammation and your gut microbiome, which are the main causative factors in the development of obesity and chronic diseases such as type 2 diabetes, fatty liver, cardiovascular disease and dental disease. This way of eating, along with regular physical activity, good sleep, reduced stress, moderate sun exposure and avoiding smoking will give you the best chance of a long and healthy life.

These are the key points to remember:

- We're too fat and have too much chronic disease – type 2 diabetes, heart disease and so on.
- We've been given the wrong dietary advice for 30 years.
- There's no need to count calories.
- Sugar, processed foods and seed (vegetable) oils are the problem.
- Healthy fats are fine, unhealthy fats are bad.
- Cholesterol is not the problem people think it is.
- Salt is not the devil either.
- We need long-term eating habits, not short-term diets.
- Nutrient density is more important than calories.
- Insulin is the fat storage hormone.
- Insulin resistance is a key factor in inflammation.

- Inflammation is the cause of most chronic disease.
- The gut microbiome plays a key role.
- Avoid sugar.
- Avoid seed (vegetable) oils.
- Avoid processed foods.
- Eat real food.
- Drink when you're thirsty.
- Restrict carbs if you're insulin resistant.
- A ketogenic diet is good for the severely insulin resistant.
- Fasting can be healthy.
- Only eat when you're hungry.
- You can find healthy food in fast-food outlets – you just have to look hard.
- Gluten sensitivity is real.
- Sweeteners aren't much better than sugar.
- You probably don't need supplements.
- Vegetarianism can be healthy with some effort.
- Eating healthily can be cheap.
- Eating out can be healthy.
- Reading food labels is a challenge.
- Good nutrition starts with kids.
- Women may have special nutrition needs.
- Exercise is a must.
- Quantity and quality of sleep are so important.
- Coping with stress requires strategies.
- Some sun exposure is necessary.
- Type 2 diabetes is reversible.
- Fatty liver can also be reversed.
- Tooth decay is a major problem among our children.
- Diet should be the first line of treatment for chronic diseases.

The Problem with Our Health System . . . and How to Fix It

We have an illness care system not a health care system

Our health system is failing us.

Despite all the advances in medical knowledge, all the new techniques, all the new drugs, all the billions of dollars we're spending on our health, we're getting fatter and sicker by the day.

If a public company performed as badly as this, the shareholders would be up in arms, the CEO would be forced to resign, and so would the board. Well, we're the shareholders in the public company known as Australia's Health, and we need to let our 'leaders' know that we want something done.

Our current health system is based on the *illness* model of health. In other words, doctors like me sit around and watch while our patients eat crap and sit on their bums until they come to us with an illness such as type 2 diabetes, and then we ply then with drugs and/or surgery to fix them, at a huge cost to the taxpayer. It's a totally inefficient and failing system.

> The World Health Organization predicts that by 2020 two thirds of all disease worldwide will be the result of lifestyle choices.

What's the alternative?

A *health*-based model of care where the emphasis is on the lifestyle issues that inevitably lead to these chronic diseases, and on making the necessary adjustments to prevent these conditions from developing. Most of the diseases we're talking about – type 2 diabetes, hypertension, coronary heart disease, stroke, Parkinson's disease, dementia, Alzheimer's disease, multiple sclerosis, and autoimmune diseases such as Crohn's disease, rheumatoid arthritis, and so on – the list goes on and on – are all largely preventable. Why are we waiting until people get sick when we know what we have to do to prevent it?

Surely all this is the fault of the medical profession. We're the ones giving out the drugs and ignoring the lifestyle issues. Yes, I know. Sometimes I'm embarrassed to be a member of my profession. But don't be too hard on the doctors.

We can be ignorant. That might surprise you. After all, doctors have five or six years' training at medical school then lots more on-the-job training, so how can they be ignorant? Doctors are taught an awful lot about treating illness – primarily with drugs and surgery. We're not taught about nutrition. We're not taught about exercise. We're not taught about the lifestyle changes necessary to prevent illness. Now I know I did my medical studies a long time ago, but I didn't have a single lecture on either nutrition or exercise. Every medical course has a subject called Pharmacology and a subject called Surgery. None of them has a subject called Nutrition or a subject called Exercise.

It's only natural to stick to the area you know. To stay in your comfort zone. Doctors are no different. They'll stick to the area they know – drugs and surgery – and avoid talking about subjects they don't understand like nutrition and exercise.

It certainly doesn't help that much of the nutrition knowledge accepted by the public is wrong, but that's one of the other faults of my profession. We're very reluctant to change, to go against what we're taught in medical school, against the accepted wisdom of the time. As a wise man once said, 'Half of everything you are taught in medical school turns out to be wrong – you just have to work out what half.'

We just assume that the accepted wisdom is based on good scientific and clinical evidence. Unfortunately, as you've seen in this book, the basis of much of the current nutrition advice, for example, was never based on scientific evidence, but rather influenced by power, ego and money. We must remember that the pharmaceutical industry (Big Pharma) and the food industry (Big Food) have billions of dollars invested in maintaining the status quo, so anyone who challenges that status quo in a way that may be detrimental to Big Pharma or Big Food is immediately challenged. Big Pharma and Big Food also have the money to influence government, both through employing large numbers of lobbyists and through regular large political donations.

Unfortunately, due to the lack of courageous political leadership in our country and many other Western countries, the government won't take the lead on these issues. It will only respond to pressure from its 'shareholders' – the electorate.

So it's up to us to demand change. If enough of us do that, the government will realise there are votes to be won in making the necessary improvements to our health. Sadly, that's their only motivation – getting themselves re-elected.

What does that change look like? Here are some of the things we can do to improve our individual health and that of the nation.

Food

Revise the *Dietary Guidelines* and Health Star Ratings to reflect the evidence that it's sugar, processed foods and vegetable oils that are killing us rather than saturated animal fats and cholesterol.

Schools

- Make the teaching of good nutrition a priority in schools.
- Improve the nutrition knowledge of teachers.
- Ban sugar-sweetened beverages from school canteens and vending machines.
- Install water fountains in schools.
- Plant a vegetable garden in every school.
- Show *That Sugar Film* at every school in the country.

Communities

- Create and maintain bike paths and running trails.
- Install water fountains.
- Encourage children to play sport by reducing costs and improving facilities.

Hospitals

- Reduce the sugar, processed foods and vegetable oils in hospital canteens and inpatient meals, and replace them with real foods.
- Remove sugar-sweetened beverages from hospital canteens and vending machines.

Workplaces

- Improve the food quality at work canteens.
- Remove sugar-sweetened beverages from work canteens and vending machines.
- Install water fountains.

Government

- Invest more in Public Health and Prevention. Australia's investment in these areas is shrinking, and we now rank in the lowest third of the OECD nations, well behind New Zealand, which leads the way at 7 per cent of total health expenditure, and Canada, second at 5.9 per cent. In 2011–12, Australian governments allocated just 1.7 per cent of total healthcare spending to public health activities, and it hasn't improved since then.
- Make preventing childhood obesity a key plank of government policy.
- Improve nutrition panel labelling by adding a category 'added sugars'.
- Bring the Health Star Rating system in line with current evidence.
- Make nutrition labelling more prominent, with larger type, and put it on the front of the pack.
- Introduce a front-of-pack label listing the amount of sugar (e.g. a picture of a teaspoon with a number denoting the number of teaspoons of sugar contained within).
- Prohibit TV advertising of unhealthy food at times when a significant number of children are likely to be watching – 6–9 a.m. and 4–9 p.m. on weekdays, and morning, afternoon and evening on weekends and school holidays.
- Pass legislation prohibiting all other forms of promoting unhealthy food to children, including via print, radio, internet, cinema, outdoor media, direct marketing (email, SMS or direct mail), product packaging or point-of-sale promotions.
- Replace sponsorship of professional and grass-roots sporting clubs.
- Implement a 20 per cent sugar tax on all foods and drinks containing significant amounts of sugar.

Doctors

- Improve education on nutrition and exercise for medical students and young doctors.
- Doctors should allow patients to educate them about healthy eating.
- Every doctor in Australia should be encouraged to read Nina Teicholz's book *The Big Fat Surprise*.

Your Toolkit

Here I'm giving you some of the tools you'll need to implement the strategies we have discussed. Firstly, it contains a selection of my favourite recipes. They are all low in sugar and avoid vegetable oils. They have good sources of proteins and contain healthy fats. Then I describe the practical ways by which we assess body fat, the background behind the blood tests commonly used to assess our heath, and give you a list of the various names used for sugar to help you identify it on food labels.

My Favourite Recipes

Doc's muesli

Serves 12 (approximately ⅓ cup per serve)

Preparation: 10 minutes
Cooking: 10 minutes

80 g (½ cup) almonds, coarsely chopped

70 g (½ cup) macadamia nuts, coarsely chopped

50 g (½ cup) walnuts, coarsely chopped

70 g (½ cup) hazelnuts, coarsely chopped

35 g (¼ cup) pistachio kernels

40 g (¼ cup) pepitas

35 g (¼ cup) sunflower seeds

50 g (1 cup) unsweetened coconut flakes

1½ teaspoons ground cinnamon

3 teaspoons vanilla bean paste

1 tablespoon flaxseeds

1 tablespoon chia seeds

1   Preheat oven to 170°C or 150°C fan forced and line a large baking tray with baking paper.
2   Place almonds, macadamias, walnuts, hazelnuts, pistachios, pepitas, sunflower seeds, coconut, cinnamon and vanilla in a large bowl. Toss until well combined.
3   Spread out evenly on prepared tray. Bake for 8–10 minutes or until light golden and crisp. Set aside to cool, stir through flaxseeds and chia seeds. Store in an airtight container for up to 3 weeks.

Tip: Can be served 'raw' or cooked, with unsweetened thick Greek yoghurt and fresh berries.

Per serve:

6.5 g protein

22.7 g fat (4.3 g saturated fat)

2.4 g carb

4.1 g dietary fibre

1022 kj (244 cals)

6 mg sodium

Big breakfast
Serves 1

Preparation: 5 minutes
Cooking: 5 minutes

3 eggs
2 teaspoons butter
1 tablespoon chopped fresh chives
20 g baby spinach leaves

50 g sliced smoked salmon
½ avocado, sliced
Lime wedge, to serve

1   Whisk the eggs together in a medium-size bowl until well combined.
2   Heat the butter in a small non-stick frying pan over medium-low heat. Pour egg mixture into pan and cook, folding occasionally, for 2 minutes or until cooked to your liking. Fold chives through scrambled eggs.
3   Serve eggs with spinach, salmon, avocado and a wedge of lime.

Per serve:
30.2 g protein
40.8 g fat (12.9 g saturated fat)
0.9 g carb
3.4 g dietary fibre
2069 kj (495 cals)
940 mg sodium

Three-seed bread
Makes 12 slices

Preparation: 10 minutes
Cooking: 40–45 minutes

50 g (⅓ cup) coconut flour
110 g (1 cup) psyllium husks
50 g (¼ cup) chia seeds
110 g (⅔ cup) pepitas (pumpkin
  seeds)
110 g (¾ cup) sunflower seeds,
  plus 2 teaspoons extra to sprinkle

1 tablespoon baking powder
½ teaspoon salt
4 eggs
350 ml (1½ cups) water
75 g unsalted butter, melted

1   Preheat oven to 180°C or 160°C fan forced. Line a 10 × 20cm (base measurement) loaf tin with baking paper, allowing the paper to overhang on the two long sides.
2   Combine flour, psyllium, chia, pepitas, sunflower seeds, baking powder and salt in a large bowl. Whisk the eggs and water together in a jug. Add to flour mixture and stir until well combined. Stir through butter.
3   Spoon mixture into prepared tin, smooth surface with the back of a spoon, sprinkle with extra sunflower seeds. Bake for 40–45 minutes or until golden and a skewer inserted into the centre comes out cleanly. Set aside to cool for 5 minutes, then transfer to a wire rack and set aside to cool completely.

Tip: This bread freezes beautifully. Cut into slices, wrap individually in plastic wrap and freeze for up to 1 month.

Per serve (slice):
8.9 g protein
17.2 g fat (5.1 g saturated fat)
4.3 g carb
10.8 g dietary fibre
946 kj (226 cals)
240 mg sodium

Bacon, feta & avocado salad

Serves 4

Preparation: 10 minutes
Cooking: 5 minutes

2 tablespoons olive oil, plus
  1 teaspoon extra
175 g middle bacon rashers,
  rind off
100 g mixed salad leaves

1 Lebanese cucumber, sliced
1 red capsicum, deseeded, sliced
1 avocado, sliced
1 tablespoon balsamic vinegar
40 g feta cheese, crumbled

1 Heat extra oil in a large non-stick frying pan over medium-high heat. Cook bacon for 2–3 minutes each side or until golden and crisp. Roughly chop.
2 Combine salad leaves, cucumber, capsicum, avocado and bacon in a large bowl. Whisk the olive oil and balsamic in a small bowl until well combined. Add dressing to salad and gently toss to combine. Serve topped with feta.

Per serve:
12.4 g protein
29.4 g fat (8.0 g saturated fat)
4.8 g carb
3.8 g dietary fibre
1419 kj (339 cals)
719 mg sodium

'Zoodle' carbonara

Serves 4

Preparation: 10 minutes
Cooking: 10 minutes

1 kg (about 8) zucchini, cut into
  'zoodles' (see tip)
½ teaspoon sea salt
3 egg yolks
2 tablespoons pure cream
40 g (½ cup) finely grated parmesan
  cheese, plus 2 tbs extra to serve

1½ tablespoons olive oil
100 g pancetta, diced
2 garlic cloves, crushed
2 tablespoons finely chopped fresh
  flat-leaf parsley

1   Place zoodles in a large colander, sprinkle with sea salt and set aside
    for 10 minutes. Rinse zoodles under cold running water. Pat dry with
    absorbent paper to remove excess moisture.
2   Whisk the egg yolks, cream and parmesan together in a medium-size
    bowl. Season with salt and pepper. Set aside.
3   Heat 2 teaspoons of the oil in a large frying pan over medium heat.
    Cook the pancetta, stirring, for 5 minutes or until golden and crisp.
    Transfer to a plate and set aside. Heat remaining oil in same pan over
    medium heat. Add garlic and cook, stirring, for 1 minute or until
    fragrant. Add zoodles and cook, tossing with tongs, for 1–2 minutes
    or until just tender. Do not overcook. Remove from heat.
4   Return pancetta to pan with egg mixture and quickly toss, until egg
    mixture coats zoodles and forms a glossy sauce. Season with salt and
    pepper. Serve immediately garnished with parsley and extra parmesan.

Tip: The easiest way to make zoodles is to use a spiraliser, available at
kitchenware stores. Alternatively, you can use a vegetable peeler to cut
zucchini into wide long strips, then use a knife to cut into thin 'zoodles'.

Tip: Salting the zucchini before cooking helps remove excess moisture and
prevents soggy 'zoodles'. It is also important not to overcook them.

Per serve:
11.8 g protein
24.6 g fat (9.0 g saturated fat)
4.8 g carb

3.2 g dietary fibre
1221 kj (292 cals)
452 mg sodium

Baked soy & sesame salmon with cauliflower rice

Serves 4

Preparation: 10 minutes
Cooking: 5 minutes

1 tablespoon sesame oil

1½ tablespoons reduced-salt soy sauce

4 × 125 g salmon fillets, skin on

600 g cauliflower, cut into florets

2½ tablespoons coconut oil

1 onion, finely chopped

1 long fresh red chilli, deseeded, finely chopped

3 garlic cloves, thinly sliced

2 teaspoons finely grated fresh ginger

2 tablespoons chopped fresh coriander

2 bunches asparagus, steamed, to serve

1   Preheat oven to 220°C or 200°C fan forced and line a baking tray with baking paper. Combine sesame oil and soy in a shallow dish. Add salmon and turn to coat. Cover and set aside to marinate for 15 minutes. Drain salmon of excess marinade and place on prepared tray. Bake for 10–12 minutes or until cooked to your liking.

2   Meanwhile, process the cauliflower in a food processor until it forms coarse crumbs (will resemble rice).

3   Heat coconut oil in a large deep non-stick frying pan or wok over medium-high heat. Cook onion, stirring, for 3–4 minutes or until softened. Add chilli, garlic and ginger and cook, stirring, for 1 minute or until fragrant. Add cauliflower and cook, stirring, for 3–4 minutes or until cauliflower is just tender. Stir through coriander.

4   Serve salmon on the cauliflower rice with steamed asparagus.

Per serve:

32.8 g protein

33.3 g fat (14.5 g saturated fat)

4.7 g carb

6.7 g dietary fibre

1927 kj (461 cals)

362 mg sodium

Zucchini, pesto & olive cauliflower crust pizza
Serves 2

Preparation: 10 minutes
Cooking: 10 minutes

500 g cauliflower florets
1 egg, lightly beaten
1 tablespoon olive oil

20 g (¼ cup) finely grated
    parmesan cheese

Topping

2 tablespoons basil pesto
1 small zucchini, thinly sliced
75 g cherry tomatoes, halved
30 g pitted black olives

40 g feta cheese, crumbled
2 tablespoons fresh basil leaves
2 teaspoons olive oil, to drizzle

1   Process the cauliflower in a food processor until it forms coarse crumbs (will resemble rice). Place in a large microwave-proof safe dish, cover, and microwave on high (100%) for 5 minutes or until just tender. Drain. Return to bowl and set aside until completely cooled.
2   Preheat oven to 220°C or 200°C fan forced. Line a large pizza tray with baking paper.
3   Add egg, 2 teaspoons oil and the parmesan to cauliflower. Press mixture into a 22cm circle on prepared pizza tray. Drizzle with remaining oil and bake for 15 minutes or until edges are golden.
4   Spread pesto evenly over base. Top with zucchini, tomatoes, olives and feta. Return to oven and bake for a further 10 minutes or until golden. Sprinkle with basil leaves and drizzle with olive oil to serve.

Tip: Recipe can easily be doubled to make 2 large pizzas to serve 4.

Per serve:
18.3 g protein
39.6 g fat (10.0 g saturated fat)
7.4 g carb
9.3 g dietary fibre
1992 kj (477 cals)
665 mg sodium

Broccoli cheese soup
Serves 4

Preparation: 10 minutes
Cooking: 10 minutes

1½ tablespoons olive oil
1 onion, finely chopped
2 garlic cloves, crushed
800 g broccoli, chopped
750 ml (3 cups) salt-reduced
   chicken stock

60 g (½ cup) grated vintage
   cheddar cheese
125 ml (½ cup) pure cream
2 tablespoons chopped fresh
   chives, to serve

1   Heat the oil in a large saucepan over medium heat. Cook the onion, stirring, for 5 minutes or until softened. Add garlic and cook, stirring, for 1 minute or until fragrant. Add broccoli and stock and bring to the boil. Reduce heat and simmer, uncovered, for 8–10 minutes or until broccoli is tender but still bright green (be careful to not overcook).

2   Set aside to cool slightly then blend soup in batches. Return soup to a clean saucepan and heat over a low heat. Add cheese and 60 ml (¼ cup) cream, stir to combine and season with black pepper. Serve with a drizzle of remaining cream, sprinkled with chives.

Tip: Soup can be frozen. Place cooled soup in individual-serve, airtight containers, cover and freeze for up to 1 month.

Per serve:
14.2 g protein
24.0 g fat (11.7 g saturated fat)
4.2 g carb
8.1 g dietary fibre
1274 kj (305 cals)
679 mg sodium

Kale, cabbage & pecan slaw

Serves 4

Preparation: 10 minutes

150 g red cabbage, shredded
75 g trimmed kale, shredded
1 red capsicum, thinly sliced
½ small red onion, thinly sliced

40 g (⅓ cup) pecan nuts, chopped
2 tablespoons extra virgin olive oil
1 tablespoon apple cider vinegar
2 teaspoons Dijon mustard

1   Combine the cabbage, kale, capsicum, onions and pecans in a large bowl.
2   Whisk the olive oil, vinegar and mustard together in a small bowl until well combined. Drizzle salad with dressing, gently toss to combine. Season with salt and pepper. Serve.

Per serve:
4.8 g protein
28.2 g fat (18.1 g saturated fat)
9.0 g carb
3.2 g dietary fibre
1324 kj (317 cals)
56 mg sodium

Berries & cream sundae
Serves 4

Preparation: 10 minutes

185 ml (¾ cup) thickened cream
1 teaspoon vanilla bean paste
125 g fresh raspberries

200 g (¾ cup) thick Greek yoghurt
250 g fresh strawberries, hulled,
  thinly sliced

1   Using electric beaters, beat cream and vanilla in a large bowl until soft
    peaks form. Place one third of the raspberries in a separate bowl and
    crush with a fork. Spoon the crushed raspberries and yoghurt through
    the cream mixture.
2   Divide cream mixture, remaining raspberries and strawberries between
    4 serving glasses. Serve.

Tip: Sundaes can be made 2–3 hours ahead, covered and refrigerated until
ready to serve.

Per serve:
4.8 g protein
28.2 g fat (18.1 g saturated fat)
9.0 g carb
3.2 g dietary fibre
1324 kj (317 cals)
56 mg sodium

Bone broth

Makes approximately 1.5 L (6 cups)

Preparation: 10 minutes
Cooking: 12–24 hours

1.5 kg chicken bones
1 onion, chopped
2 carrots, peeled, chopped
3 sticks celery, chopped
2 garlic cloves, peeled

1 tablespoon olive oil
1 teaspoon salt
2 bay leaves
1 teaspoon black peppercorns

1   Preheat oven to 200°C or 180°C fan forced. Place chicken bones, onion, carrots, celery and garlic in a large baking dish. Drizzle with olive oil and sprinkle with salt. Bake for 30 minutes or until browned.
2   Transfer bones and vegetables to a slow cooker. Add 2 L (8 cups) water, the bay leaves and peppercorns. Cook on low for 12–24 hours. Set aside to cool.
3   Strain through a fine sieve, discard solids.

Tip: To freeze, divide broth between airtight containers, cover and freeze for up to 2 months.

Tip: Chicken carcasses are ideal to use and can be purchased from your local butcher; you will need 2–3 carcasses. For beef bone broth, substitute the chicken bones with oxtail. At the end of the cooking time, strain and shred any meat from the oxtail. This meat can then be added to soups or stews.

Home-made tomato sauce

Makes approximately 400 ml (12 serves)

Preparation: 10 minutes
Cooking: 20 minutes

2½ tablespoons olive oil
1 onion, finely chopped
2 garlic cloves, crushed
½ teaspoon smoked paprika

¼ teaspoon allspice
400 ml tomato purée
1 tablespoon red wine vinegar

1   Heat the oil in a large saucepan over medium heat. Cook onion, stirring, for 5 minutes or until softened. Add garlic, paprika and all-spice and cook, stirring, for 1 minute or until fragrant.
2   Add tomato purée and vinegar and bring to the boil. Reduce heat to low and simmer, partially covered, for 12–15 minutes or until thickened. Season with salt and pepper.
3   Set aside to cool. Blend in a blender or food processor until smooth.

Tip: Sauce can be frozen in small airtight containers for up to 3 months or will keep covered in the fridge for 3–4 days.

Per serve:
0.8 g protein
3.9 g fat (0.6 g saturated fat)
2.0 g carb
0.7 g dietary fibre
200 kj (48 cals)
77 mg sodium

How to Measure Body Fat

Definitions of overweight and obesity have always been based on body mass index (BMI) results.

BMI is:

$$\text{Weight in kilograms}/(\text{Height in metres})^2$$

So if you weigh 80 kilograms and are 1.80 metres tall, your BMI is:

$$80/1.8^2 = 80/3.24 = 24.7$$

There are many online calculators, such as this one: healthyweight.health.gov.au/wps/portal/Home/helping-hand/bmi.

What your BMI tells you

Weight category	BMI
Underweight	<18.5
Normal	18.5–24.9
Overweight	25.0–29.9
Obesity I	30.0–34.9
Obesity II	35.0–39.9
Extreme obesity III	>40.0

BMI levels are the most commonly used measure of obesity, but they have their limitations, especially in men with large muscle mass and people with non-Caucasian ancestry.

More accurate measures of body fat

Body fat percentage is more precise than BMI. There are a number of methods of calculating body fat percentage.

1. DEXA (dual-energy X-ray absorptiometry) scan

This total body scan is used more commonly to measure bone density but also measures fat and muscle mass. It's the most accurate but also the most expensive method!

2. Bioelectrical impedance analysis devices (BIA)

Bioelectrical impedance analysis (BIA) measures the body's resistance to a light electrical current. These are cheaper and quicker than DEXA scans, but are not as accurate.

3. Skin calipers

In skinfold testing, skin calipers are used to pinch the skin and the subcutaneous fat (fat underneath the skin), pull the skinfold away from the underlying muscle, and measure its thickness.

Skin calipers can be used at a single site or a sum of skinfolds can be performed. This is commonly used by fitness personnel working with sporting teams, and as long as the same person is doing the measuring, they're reasonably accurate at detecting changes in body fat.

4. Bathroom scales

Old-fashioned, but still a pretty good indication, certainly of progressive weight loss (or gain).

5. Waist measurement

Measure your waist circumference with a tape measure. Place the tape measure directly on your skin, halfway between your lowest rib and the top of your hip bone, roughly in line with your belly button. Breathe out normally and measure.

This measurement can be used in a number of ways:

Waist circumference

Waist circumference thresholds indicating increased risk of disease are:

	Waist circumference for . . .	
Gender	Increased disease risk	High disease risk
Female	≥80 cm	≥88 cm
Male	≥94 cm	≥102 cm for men

Waist-to-hip ratio (WHR)

Measure waist circumference as above. Measure hip circumference at their widest point, usually at the top of the hip bone. Divide your waist measurement by your hip measurement or use an online calculator, such as www.mydr.com.au/tools/waist-to-hip-calculator.

Excess abdominal fat distribution is indicated by a WHR greater than 0.8 for women and 0.9 for men.

Waist-to-height (WH) ratio

A recent study suggested that the WH ratio was more accurate than BMI at predicting the percentage of body fat.[1] Divide your waist measurement by your height (make sure they're both in the same units – i.e. your height is in centimetres rather than metres) or use an online calculator, such as www.health-calc.com/body-composition/waist-to-height-ratio.

A ratio of more than 0.53 in men and 0.54 in women is a predictor of whole-body obesity. Greater than 0.59 in either sex is a predictor of abdominal obesity.

What Blood Tests
Should I Have?

Blood tests can give a good indication of how healthy you are. Here's a run-down of the blood tests that will give you the most valuable information about your health.

Full blood count

A full blood count (FBC) provides a lot of information. The main components are:

- haemoglobin (Hb): <130 (men) and <115 (women) indicates anaemia
- white blood cell count (WCC): >10 indicates presence of infection
- platelet count: generally <400 – important in blood clotting

Lipids

The standard lipid profile consists of:

- Total cholesterol: should be <5.0 mmol/L
- LDL cholesterol: should be <4.0 mmol/L
- HDL cholesterol: should be >1.0 mmol/L
- Triglycerides: should be <1.5 mmol/L
- Total cholesterol to HDL cholesterol ratio: should be <5

As you know, I believe the two important components of the lipid profile are the triglyceride and HDL cholesterol levels. For your triglyceride to HDL ratio, simply divide your triglyceride level by your HDL level:

Triglycerides = 1.5, HDL = 1.0, so Trig/HDL ratio = 1.5/1.0 = 1.5

As I said, I like that ratio to be under 1.5. There are also online calculators, such as www.hughcalc.org/chol-si.php.

Diabetes

Several blood tests are used in the diagnosis of type 2 diabetes:

- **Fasting blood glucose (FBG)**: should be <5.5 mmol/L. This has traditionally been the standard test for diabetes, with levels higher than 5.5 mmol/L diagnosed as diabetes.
- **HbA1c**: should be <5.6 per cent. This gives a better indication of blood glucose over the preceding three months. The normal range for the haemoglobin A1c level is 4–5.6 per cent. HbA1c levels of 5.7–6.4 per cent mean you have a higher change of developing diabetes. Levels of 6.5 per cent or higher mean you already have diabetes. The HbA1c is also used to monitor levels in those already diagnosed as diabetic.
- **Serum insulin**: should be <9 μIU/ml. This isn't part of the standard diabetes tests, but it's very useful for detecting hyperinsulinemia (high blood insulin), an important early indicator of insulin resistance.

Liver function tests (LFTs)

Fatty liver does not cause any particular symptoms until it's well advanced. It is, however, associated with abdominal obesity – the so-called apple shape – rather than the pear shape, where most of the fat is around the buttocks and thighs. The presence of a 'sugar' belly, where your waist is larger than your hips, should make you concerned that you could have a fatty liver. Fatty liver is often associated with high blood triglyceride levels, so if yours are, you should ask for a liver function test.

Fatty liver is first recognised on the basis of blood tests known as liver function tests. These measure a number of enzymes that are elevated in fatty liver, such as ALT and GGT (you don't need to know their full names).

The standard LFTs are:

- bilirubin
- ALP (alkaline phosphatase)
- GGT (gamma-glutamyl transferase)
- AST (aspartate transaminase)
- ALT (alanine transaminase).

The best indicators of fatty liver are raised GGT and ALT levels.

Inflammation

C-reactive protein (CRP) and erythrocyte sedimentation rate (ESR) are non-specific markers of inflammation, which as we have discussed is associated with most chronic diseases. CRP should be <3 mg/dL, and ESR <20 mm/h.

More recently, a newer, more sensitive CRP test – high-sensitivity CRP – has been found useful in identifying those at increased risk of CVD. C-reactive protein (hsCRP) adds prognostic information on cardiovascular risk comparable to blood pressure or cholesterol. Values <1, 1 to 3, and >3 mg/l indicate lower, average or higher relative cardiovascular risk, respectively. Each standard deviation increase in hsCRP is associated with a 37 per cent increase in risk of coronary heart disease – an effect at least as large as those reported for total cholesterol, high-density lipoprotein cholesterol (HDL-C), and blood pressure. Importantly, hsCRP levels track with the severity and number of underlying features of metabolic syndrome, and predict vascular risk among those already defined as having significant insulin resistance.

hsCRP testing is available locally and is appropriate in primary prevention settings such as when a clinical decision to initiate statin therapy is uncertain, or for monitoring the effect of lifestyle and diet changes on risk.[1]

Vitamin D

Vitamin D deficiency is thought to be a risk factor for a number of medical conditions. As we have seen, there's considerable debate about what level of vitamin D constitutes deficiency.

Deficiency status	Vitamin D level (nmol/L)
Severely deficient	<30
Deficient	<50
Sub-optimal	<80
Ideal	>80

Iron and B12 studies

If you're vegetarian or vegan, it's important to monitor your iron and B12 levels. Iron studies in blood tests consist of:

- serum iron: should be 12–32 μmol/L
- total iron binding capacity (TIBC): should be 45–66 μmol/L
- transferrin saturation: should be 20–50 per cent
- serum ferritin: should be 30–150 μg/L in women, and 50–250 μg/L in men.

Serum ferritin is a measure of iron stores. The labs tell you that less than 15–20 μg/L is abnormal, but I believe that levels less than 50 μg/L are indicative of insufficient iron stores and may specifically impair athletic performance.

Vitamin B12 levels should be >200 pmol/L. Some think that any B12 level under 500 pmol/L is indicative of deficiency and should be treated.

Other Names for Sugar

Sugars	Syrups	Technical names	The rest
Barbados sugar	Agave syrup	Carbohydrate	Agave (including nectar)
Beet sugar	Barley malt syrup	blend	Applesauce
Blonde coconut	Birch syrup	Crystal fructose	Banana
sugar	Brown rice syrup	Crystalline fructose	Barley malt
Brown sugar	Buttered syrup	Crystalline sucrose	Biodynamic raisins
Buttered sugar	Cane syrup	Dextran	Cane juice (including
Cane sugar	(including	Dextrose	crystals, dehydrated,
Caster sugar	dehydrated,	Diatase	solids)
Coco sap sugar	organic)	Diastatic malt	Caramel
Coco sugar	Carob syrup	Ethyl maltol	Carob
Coconut palm	Coconut syrup	Fructose (including	Coconut blossom
sugar	Corn syrup	crystals)	Coconut nectar (including
Coconut sugar	(including light,	Galactose	dehydrated, palm
Confectioner's	organic)	Glucose	nectar)
sugar	Corn syrup solids	Glucose solids	Corn sweetener
Date sugar	Golden syrup	Lactose	Dates (including medjool,
Demerara sugar	High fructose	Maltitol	paste)
Free-flowing brown	corn syrup (aka	Maltodextrin	Evaporated cane juice
sugar	HFCS)	Maltol	Fig paste
Golden sugar	Invert syrup	Maltose	Florida crystals
Grape sugar	Lucuma syrup	Mannose	Fruit juice (including
Icing sugar	Malt syrup	Saccharose	concentrate, crystals)
Malt sugar	Maple syrup	Sucrose	Fruit purée
Maple sugar	Molasses syrup		Honey (including organic,
Muscovado sugar	Oat syrup		raw, Manuka)
Organic	Pure maple syrup		Jaggery
dehydrated cane	Rice bran syrup		Mascobado/muscovado
sugar	Rice malt syrup		Molasses (including
Organic raw sugar	Rice syrup		blackstrap, dry cane,
Palm sugar	Sorghum syrup		unsulfured)
Powdered sugar	Syrup		Nectar
Rapadura sugar	Tapioca syrup		Panocha
Raw sugar	Yacon syrup		Pure cane
Refiner's sugar			Raisin juice concentrate
Sugar			Raw blue agave
Table sugar			Raw coconut crystals
Turbinado sugar			Sucanat
Yellow sugar			Sweet sorghum
			Treacle
			Turbinado (including
			natural)
			White grape juice
			concentrate

Resources

If you want to learn more about the many topics I've covered in this book, there are lots of good resources. I've listed my Top Tens here under five categories: movies, books, YouTube videos, websites/blogs and podcasts. For a full list of resources, see fatlotofgood.com.au.

Movies

1 *That Sugar Film* (2015)
thatsugarfilm.com
Damon Gameau ate only foods commonly thought to be healthy or promoted that way, and in the process documented the effects of a high-sugar diet. Clever. Funny. The whole family should watch it.

2 *Cereal Killers 1* (2013)
www.cerealkillersmovie.com
Tim Noakes gets Donal O'Neill started on his low-carb journey. Featuring cameos from some Aussie cricketers and their doctor (no names mentioned!).

3 *Cereal Killers 2: Run on Fat* (2015)
www.runonfatmovie.com
Triathlete Sami Inkinen and his wife Meredith undertake to row 6400 kilometres from San Francisco to Hawaii fuelled by fat and advised by Steve Phinney. Remarkable story.

4 *Cereal Killers 3: The Big Fat Fix* (2016)
www.thebigfatfix.com
Donal O'Neill and cardiologist Aseem Malhotra visit the citizens of the tiny Italian village of Pioppi to find out the secret of their longevity.

5 *Fed Up* (2014)
www.fedupmovie.com
Filmmaker Stephanie Soechtig and journalist Katie Couric investigate the American food industry and whether it's responsible for more sickness than we thought.

6 *The Magic Pill: Food Is Medicine* (2017)
fan-force.com/films/themagicpill
Pete Evans looks at doctors, patients, scientists, chefs, farmers and journalists from around the world who are embracing fat as fuel and combating disease.

7 *Carb-Loaded: A Culture Dying to Eat* (2015)

carbloaded.com

Looks at the reasons behind the rise in diabetes over the past 30 years, and what we can do about it. It features interviews with lots of interesting people in the low-carb world.

8 *Fat Chance* (2017)

This documentary follows Warren Hepworth, who sets out to ride a bike from Perth to Melbourne on a low-carbohydrate, high-fat diet. Beware – there are a number of movies called *Fat Chance*!

9 *Fat Head* (2009)

www.fathead-movie.com

Stand-up comedian Tom Naughton tries to lose weight on a fast-food diet and prove Morgan Spurlock (of *Super Size Me* fame) wrong. He soon realises he's been wrong himself in focusing only on calories.

10 *Fixing Dad* (2015)

www.fixingdad.com

In this BBC doco two brothers help their dad change from an obese night-time security guard barely able to move to an endurance cyclist, health activist and public speaker.

Books

1 *The Big Fat Surprise* (2014) by Nina Teicholz
2 *Good Calories, Bad Calories* (2007) by Gary Taubes
3 *What the Fat?* (2015) by Grant Schofield, Caryn Zinn & Craig Rodger
4 *The Real Meal Revolution* (2015) by Tim Noakes, Sally-Ann Creed, Jonno Proudfoot & David Grier
5 *The Pioppi Diet* (2017) by Aseem Malhotra & Donal O'Neill
6 *The Obesity Epidemic* (2010) by Zoë Harcombe
7 *The Obesity Code* (2016) by Jason Fung
8 *Fat Chance* (2012) by Robert H. Lustig
9 *The Art and Science of Low Carbohydrate Living* (2011) by Jeff S. Volek & Stephen D. Phinney
10 *Fat Is Our Friend* (2016) by Sammy Pepys

YouTube videos

1 'Sugar: The Bitter Truth' with Robert Lustig, www.youtube.com/watch?v=dBnniua6-oM
2 'Tim Noakes – UCT Faculty of Health Sciences Centenary Debate' with Tim Noakes, www.youtube.com/watch?v=5IYVIdztWWs

3 'Medical Aspects of the Low Carbohydrate Lifestyle' with Tim Noakes, www. youtube.com/watch?v=fL5-9ZxamXc

4 'Toxic Sugar', ABC TV's *Catalyst*, www.youtube.com/watch?v=UU3GvRsFHqY

5 'The Food Revolution' with Andreas Eenfeldt, www.youtube.com/watch?v= FSeSTq-N4U4

6 'Reversing Type 2 Diabetes Starts with Ignoring the Guidelines' with Sarah Hallberg, TEDxPurdueU, www.youtube.com/watch?v=da1vvigy5tQ

7 'How to Make Diseases Disappear' with Rangan Chatterjee, TEDx Liverpool, www.youtube.com/watch?v=gaY4m00wXpw

8 'Intermittent Fasting for Weight Loss' with Jason Fung, www.youtube.com/ watch?v=v9Aw0P7GjHE

9 'On High-Fat, Low-Carb Diets & Diabetes' with Richard Bernstein, www.you-tube.com/watch?v=vyOI9bk3VZc

10 'Why We Get Fat' with Gary Taubes, www.youtube.com/watch?v= lDneyrETR2o

Websites/blogs

1 **Diet Doctor**, www.dietdoctor.com
The biggest and best low-carb site in the world. Founded in 2011 after Swedish beginnings in 2007, Dr Andreas Eenveldt's site now has 14 full-time workers; about 20 freelancers, moderators and partners; and more than 200 000 visits per day. Great videos featuring lots of well-known presenters, articles, case studies, recipes, and so on.

2 **Ditch the Carbs**, www.ditchthecarbs.com
Libby is a Kiwi mum of three young children and a registered pharmacist who had the choice between becoming a dietitian or starting a website. Fortunately for all of us, she chose the latter. Great site full of stories, articles and high-quality infographics. Good information for families. Very practical.

3 **Nutrition Advance**, nutritionadvance.com
Michael Joseph is a nutrition educator who has put together a wonderful web-site full of high-quality content in an easy-to-read format. He does a great job of translating science into simple lessons.

4 **Eating Academy**, eatingacademy.com
Dr Peter Attia is a former elite ultra-endurance athlete who discovered nutri-tion late in his career and now has an excellent website covering nutrition and performance issues, much of it from his personal experience.

5 **Dr Mercola**, www.mercola.com
Although this site is often criticised as being 'too commercial', I still find it full of great information on a wide range of issues, including nutrition, exercise and lifestyle.

6 **Protein Power**, proteinpower.com

Michael and Mary Dan Eades, the authors of *Protein Power*, have a good website. Michael's blogs are always worth reading.

7 **Zoë Harcombe**, www.zoeharcombe.com

I love Zoë Harcombe's regular blogs. Her analysis of others' research is always insightful, and she can detect bulls. . .t from a great distance.

8 **Malcolm Kendrick**, www.drmalcolmkendrick.org

Malcolm Kendrick writes a fascinating blog unravelling the mystery of what causes heart disease.

9 **Livin La Vida Low Carb**, livinlavidalowcarb.com

Jimmy Moore is quite a character. Passionate about low-carb diets, he interviews all the big names on his podcasts and blogs.

10 **SugarByHalf**, www.sugarbyhalf.com

Bit biased here, but the SugarByHalf website has lots of good stuff, including plenty of sugar swaps.

Podcasts

1 Livin La Vida Low Carb with Jimmy Moore, livinlavidalowcarb.com/blog/tag/podcast

2 2 Keto Dudes with Carl Franklin & Richard Morris, 2ketodudes.com

3 The Paleo Solution with Robb Wolf, robbwolf.com/category/podcasts

4 Just Below Their Purpose with Sam Loy & Clint Greagen, justbelowtheirpurpose.libsyn.com

5 180 Nutrition Podcasts with Guy Lawrence & Stu Cooke, 180nutrition.com.au/180-tv-guests

6 Low Carb Conversations with Leah Williamson & Kara Halderman, www.lowcarbconversations.com

7 Ketogeek podcast, ketogeek.com

8 The Low Carb Leader with Dan Perryman, thelowcarbleader.com

9 The Keto Diet Podcast with Leanne Vogel, healthfulpursuit.com/podcast

10 Keto Talk with Jimmy Moore & Will Cole, ketotalk.com

Apps

For an updated list of useful apps for mindfulness, eating, sleeping, exercising and giving up smoking, see my website, fatlotofgood.com.au.

SugarByHalf

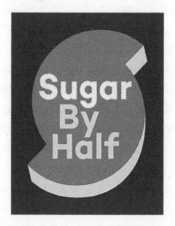

A couple of years ago I gave a talk about nutrition at a TedMed conference in Melbourne. Afterwards, I was chatting to the chair of the conference session, Dr Mei Ling Doery. I was bemoaning the fact that we weren't getting any traction with a really important message: that to solve the problems of obesity and diabetes, we need to change the way we eat.

One of the issues, I suggested to Mei, was that we had created a state of confusion about what we should be eating. For many years we'd followed the low-fat mantra, but it wasn't working. Various people were passionately advocating various diets – paleo, LCHF, Atkins, Mediterranean and more – but all we were doing was confusing people.

Wouldn't it be great, I said to Mei, if all these groups could get together and campaign on one thing – and the one thing that everyone agreed on was sugar. We all knew that sugar was a key factor in the development of these health issues. With Mei's encouragement, I set out to speak to as many people as I could over the following weeks to ascertain if there was support for a campaign to reduce sugar. I was overwhelmed by the enthusiasm of everyone I spoke to about mounting a campaign to reduce sugar intake.

And so SugarByHalf was born: with the aim of reducing the average daily intake of added sugars by half. The current average intake is around 16 teaspoons of added sugar per day, and considerably higher among teenagers in particular. The World Health Organization has indicated that about 6 teaspoons a day is ideal, so reducing our intake by a half will get us close. There's no doubt that were we to be successful and reduce the intake of added sugar by half, it would have a massive impact on the health of our country. I can think of no other intervention that would have such a dramatic effect.

At SugarByHalf we have a great group of committed people determined to do everything we can to overcome what we've called the 'sugardemic'. We launched SugarByHalf in October 2016 with a media blitz including a Facebook Live event with the support of a host of doctors, sports stars and celebrities. Since then we've been busy on social media, and speaking to groups around the country, to gain support.

The first stage of our campaign has been to increase awareness of the sugardemic and what we can do about it. We are now working on developing a community-based program to combat obesity and chronic disease.

We'll continue to educate and advocate with the goal of reducing our sugar intake.

All royalties from this book are donated to the SugarByHalf campaign.

www.sugarbyhalf.com

Acknowledgements

I couldn't have written *A Fat Lot of Good* without the help of many people.

I would firstly like to thank everyone at Penguin Random House for having belief in me and encouraging me to undertake this project. Special thanks to my editor Izzy Yates who was infinitely patient with my missed deadlines and stubborn insistence on including various aspects. Thank you to my daughter Julia Brukner for her assistance in establishing my website www.fatlotofgood.com.au.

Thank you to my friend Shane Watson for writing a kind and generous foreword. Many friends and colleagues have reviewed part or all of the book and given me valuable feedback. Thanks to Jamie Hayes, Feng-Yuan Liu, David and Pauline Eccleston, Mary Barson, Malcolm and Kathryn Kemp, Rod Tayler, Tania Sincock, Caroline Nicolson, Karim Khan, Matt Hopcraft, Darren Burgess, Ayesha Carrim, Keith De Souza, Larissa Trease and Rob Moodie.

I would also like to thank Libby Jenkinson from DitchTheCarbs, Jason Fung, Zoë Harcombe, Troy Stapleton and Matt Hopcraft for allowing me to use some of their material.

My past six years has been a wonderful journey of learning and I have met so many people who have helped enlighten me along the way. Thanks to my teachers Tim Noakes, Gary Taubes, Nina Teicholz, Aseem Malhotra, Robert Lustig, Jeff Gerber, Jason Fung, Grant Schofield, Caryn Zinn, Zoë Harcombe, Joseph Kraft, Ivor Cummins, Donal O'Neill, Adreas Eenfeldt, Malcolm Kendrick, William Davis, David Perlmutter, James DiNicolantonio, Sarah Hallberg, Catherine Shanahan, David Gillespie, Gary and Beinda Fettke, Rod Tayler, Weston A. Price, Richard Bernstein, Eric Westman, Natasha Campbell-McBride, Stephen Phinney, Jeff Volek, Fred Kummerow, Travis Christofferson, Thomas Seyfried, Terry Wahls and numerous others. You have been courageous leaders in inspiring the rest of us to to join the rapidly expanding group of health professionals who realise that lifestyle modifications are the key to good health.

Last but by no means least, thank you to my family – Diana, Julia and Sam (and Teddy), Charlie, Joe, Bill and Abs – for tolerating my obsession with this cause over the past six years, and apologies for boring you all with my sermons. I am very fortunate to have such a wonderful, supportive family.

Notes

I. The State of the Nation
Where We're At

1. Australian Institute of Health and Welfare 2016, *Australia's health 2016: in brief*, AIHW: Canberra, Cat. no. AUS 201. https://www.aihw.gov.au/reports/australias-health/australias-health-2016-in-brief/contents/are-we-a-healthy-nation.
2. Yang L. and Colditz G.A., 'Prevalence of overweight and obesity in the United States, 2007–2012', *JAMA Intern Med*, 2015, 175(8): 1412–3.
3. Australian Institute of Health and Welfare 2016, *Australia's health 2016: in brief*.
4. Australian Bureau of Statistics, 'Table 8.3', *National Health Survey: First Results, 2014–15*, Canberra: ABS, 2015. http://www.abs.gov.au/ausstats/abs@.nsf/mf/4364.0.55.001.
5. OECD, *Health at a Glance 2017: OECD Indicators*, Paris: OECD Publishing, 2017. http://dx.doi.org/10.1787/health_glance-2017-en.
6. Wade, M., 'The true cost of obesity', *Sydney Morning Herald*, 5 December 2015. www.smh.com.au/national/health/the-true-cost-of-fat-obesity-a-130-billion-drag-on-our-wellbeing-20151204-glfh6a.html.
7. Hayes A., Chevalier A., D'Souza M., et al. 'Early childhood obesity: Association with healthcare expenditure in Australia', *Obesity*, 2016, 24(8): 1752–8.
8. World Obesity, 'World Obesity Day 2017'. http://www.obesityday.worldobesity.org
9. Withrow D. and Alter D.A., 'The economic burden of obesity worldwide: a systematic review of the direct costs of obesity', *Obes Rev*, 2011, 12(2): 131–41.
10. 'How Deadly Is Obesity, Really?', *Six Minutes*, 5 September 2017. https://www.6minutes.com.au/news/how-deadly-obesity-really.
11. Australian Bureau of Statistics, 'Diabetes Mellitus', *National Health Survey: First Results, 2014–15*, Canberra: ABS, 2015. http://www.abs.gov.au/ausstats/abs@.nsf/Lookup/by%20Subject/4364.0.55.001~2014-15~Main%20Features~Diabetes%20mellitus~12.
12. Diabetes Australia, 'Diabetes in Australia'. https://www.diabetesaustralia.com.au/diabetes-in-australia.
13. American Heart Association, *Statistical Fact Sheet 2014 Update*, 2014. https://www.heart.org/idc/groups/heart-public/@wcm/@sop/@smd/documents/downloadable/ucm_462019.pdf.
14. Deloitte Access Economics, *The Economic Cost and Health Burden of Liver Disease in Australia*, January 2013. https://static1.squarespace.com/static/

50ff0804e4b007d5a9abe0a5/t/53321aaee4b09f967eb0c7e5/1395792558684/
gesa2013_revised%5B1%5D.pdf.

15. Ibid.

16. Sugar-free Smiles. sugarfreesmiles.com.

17. Australian Institute of Health and Welfare, 'Heart, stroke & vascular diseases', 2017. https://www.aihw.gov.au/reports-statistics/health-conditions-disability-deaths/heart-stroke-vascular-diseases/overview.

18. Australian Bureau of Statistics, 'Hypertension and measured high blood pressure', *National Health Survey: First Results, 2014–15*, Canberra: ABS, 2015. http://www.abs.gov.au/ausstats/abs@.nsf/Lookup/by%20Subject/4364.0.55.001~2014-15~Main%20Features~Hypertension%20and%20measured%20high%20blood%20pressure~14?opendocument&ref=stor.

19. Australian Institute of Health and Welfare 2016, *Australia's Health 2016*, AIHW: Canberra, Cat. no. AUS 199. www.aihw.gov.au/reports/australias-health/australias-health-2016/contents/ill-health.

20. Australian Bureau of Statistics, *National Health Survey: First Results, 2014–15*.

21. Dementia Australia, 'Statistics: Key facts and statistics 2017', December 2017. https://www.dementia.org.au/statistics.

22. Cancer Council Australia, 'Facts and Figures: Cancer in Australia', February 2017. http://www.cancer.org.au/about-cancer/what-is-cancer/facts-and-figures.html.

23. Australian Bureau of Statistics, *National Health Survey: First Results, 2014–15*.

24. Lawrence, D., Johnson, S., Hafekost, J., et al., *The Mental Health of Children and Adolescents. Report on the second Australian Child and Adolescent Survey of Mental Health and Wellbeing*, Department of Health: Canberra, 2015. www.health.gov.au/internet/main/publishing.nsf/content/9DA8CA21306FE6EDCA257E2700016945/$File/child2.pdf.

25. Access Economics for Arthritis Australia, *Painful Realities: The Economic Impact of Arthritis in Australia 2007*, Arthritis Australia Sydney: Sydney, 2007. www.arthritisaustralia.com.au/images/stories/documents/reports/2011_updates/painful realities report access economics.pdf.

26. World Health Organisation (WHO), 'Health Topics: Global burden of disease'. http://www.who.int/topics/global_burden_of_disease/en/.

27. GBD 2013 Risk Factors Collaborators, 'Global, regional, and national comparative risk assessment of 79 behavioural, environmental and occupational, and metabolic risks or clusters of risks in 188 countries, 1990–2013: a systematic analysis for the Global Burden of Disease Study 2013', *Lancet*, 2015, 386(10010): 2287–2323. http://doi.org/10.1016/S0140-6736(15)00128-2.

28. Australian Bureau of Statistics, *Australian Health Survey: Nutrition First Results – Foods and Nutrients, 2011–12*, ABS: Canberra, 2014. http://www.abs.gov.au/ausstats/abs@.nsf/Lookup/by%20Subject/4364.0.55.007~2011-12~Main%20Features~Discretionary%20foods~700.

29. Australian Bureau of Statistics, *Australian Health Survey: Nutrition First Results – Foods and Nutrients, 2014–15*, ABS: Canberra, 2015. http://www.abs.gov.au/ausstats/abs@.nsf/Lookup/by%20Subject/4364.0.55.001~2014-15~Main%20Features~Daily%20intake%20of%20fruit%20and%20vegetables~28.

30. Australian Bureau of Statistics, *Australian Health Survey: Consumption of added sugars, 2011–12*, ABS: Canberra, 2016. http://www.abs.gov.au/ausstats/abs@.nsf/Lookup/4364.0.55.011main+features12011-12.

31. Australian Institute of Health and Welfare, 'Risk factors to health', AIHW: Canberra, August 2017. https://www.aihw.gov.au/reports/biomedical-risk-factors/risk-factors-to-health/contents/insufficient-physical-activity.

32. Australian Institute of Health and Welfare, 'Risk factors to health', AIHW: Canberra, August 2017.

II. How Did We Get It So Wrong?
Fat Versus Sugar

1. Yudkin, J., *Pure, White and Deadly*, London: Davis-Poynter, 1972.

2. Teicholz, N., *The Big Fat Surprise: Why Butter, Meat and Cheese Belong in a Healthy Diet*, Simon & Schuster: New York, 2014.

3. Keys, A., 'Atherosclerosis: a problem in newer public health', *J Mt Sinai Hosp NY*, 1953, 20(2): 118–39.

4. Yerushalmy, J., Hilleboe, H.E., 'Fat in the diet and mortality from heart disease; a methodologic note', *N Y State J Med*, 1957, 57(14): 2343–54.

5. Keys, A., 'Coronary heart disease in seven countries. Summary', *Circulation*, 1970, 41(I-186-I-195).

6. Page, I.H., Allen, E.V., Chamberlain, F.L., Keys, A., et al., 'Dietary fat and its relation to heart attacks and strokes: Report by the Central Committee for Medical and Community Program of the AHA', *JAMA*, 1961, 175: 389–91.

7. Select Committee on Nutrition and Human Needs, US Senate, *Dietary Guidelines for the United States*, US Government Printing Office: Washington, DC, 1977. archive.org/details/CAT10527234.

8. Quoted in Taubes, G., *The Diet Delusion*, London: Vermilion, 2009, 47.

9. Ibid, 47.

10. Idem, 48.

11. Ubell, E., 'Sugar: moot factor in heart disease', *New York Herald Tribune*, 11 July 1965.

12. Select Committee on Nutrition and Human Needs, US Senate, *Dietary Guidelines for the United States*.

13. McGandy, R.B., Hegsted, D.M., Stare, F.J., et al., 'Dietary fats, carbohydrates and atherosclerotic vascular disease', *New Eng J Med*, 1967, 277(5): 186–92 and 245–47.

14. Kearns, C.E., Apollonio, D., Glantz, S., 'Sugar industry sponsorship of germ-free rodent studies linking sucrose to hyperlipidemia and cancer: An historical analysis of internal documents', *PLoS Biol*, 2017, 15(11): e2003460.

15. Mann, G., 'A short history of the diet/heart hypothesis' in George V. Mann (ed.), *Coronary Heart Disease: The Dietary Sense and Nonsense*, Janus: London, 1993, 1.

16. Ramsden, C.E., Zamora, D., Majchrzak-Hong, S., 'Re-evaluation of the traditional diet–heart hypothesis: analysis of recovered data from Minnesota Coronary Experiment (1968–73)', *BMJ*, 2016, 353: i1246.

17. Woodhill, J.M., Palmer, A.J., Leelarthaepin, B., et al., 'Low fat, low cholesterol diet in secondary prevention of coronary heart disease', *Adv Exp Med Biol*, 1978, 109: 317–30.

18. Ramsden, C.E., Zamora, D., Leelarthaepin, B., et al., 'Use of dietary linoleic acid for secondary prevention of coronary heart disease and death: evaluation of recovered data from the Sydney Diet Heart Study and updated meta-analysis', *BMJ*, 2013, 346: e8707.

19. Kmietowicz, Z., 'Coca-Cola funded group set up to promote "energy balance" is disbanded', *BMJ*, 2015, 351: h6590.

20. Harcombe, Z., 'Dietary fat guidelines have no evidence base: where next for public health nutritional advice?', *Br J Sports Med*, 2017, 51: 769–774.

21. Fernandez, M.L., Calle, M., 'Revisiting dietary cholesterol recommendations: does the evidence support a limit of 300 mg/d?', *Curr Atheroscler Rep*, 2010, 12(6): 377–83.

22. Hamley, S., 'The Effect of Replacing Saturated Fat with Mostly N-6 Poly-unsaturated Fat on Coronary Heart Disease: A Meta-Analysis of Randomised Controlled Trials', *Nutrition Journal*, 2017, 16(1): 30.

23. Ibid; and Djousse, L., Gaziano, J.M., 'Dietary cholesterol and coronary artery disease: a systematic review', *Curr Atheroscler Rep*, 2009, 11(6): 418–22.

Cholesterol: Bad Boy or Innocent Bystander?

1. Rosch, P. J., 'Cholesterol does not cause coronary heart disease in contrast to stress', *Scand Cardiovasc J*, 2008, 42(4): 244–9.

2. Gaziano, J. M., Hennekens, C. H., O'Donnell, C. J., et al., 'Fasting triglycerides, high-density lipoprotein, and risk of myocardial infarction', *Circulation*, 1997, 96: 2520–2525.

3. Kendrick, M., *The Great Cholesterol Con: The Truth About What Really Causes Heart Disease and How to Avoid It*, John Blake: London, 2007.

4. Harcombe, Z., 'Cholesterol & heart disease – there is a relationship, but it's not what you think', 23 November 2010, www.zoeharcombe.com/2010/11/cholesterol-heart-disease-there-is-a-relationship-but-its-not-what-you-think.

5. Grasgruber, P., Sebera, M., Hrazdira, E., et al., 'Food consumption and the actual statistics of cardiovascular diseases: an epidemiological comparison of 42 European countries', *Food Nutr Res*, 2016, 60: 31694.

Salt: Too Much or Too Little?

1. Dahl, L.K., Love, R.A., 'Evidence for relationship between sodium (chloride) intake and human essential hypertension', *AMA Arch Intern Med*, 1954, 94(4): 525–3.

2. Heart Foundation (Australia), 'Salt'. www.heartfoundation.org.au/healthy-eating/food-and-nutrition/salt.

3. O'Donnell, M., Mente, A., Rangarajan, S., et al., 'Urinary sodium and potassium excretion, mortality, and cardiovascular events', *N Engl J Med*, 2014, 371: 612–623; O'Donnell, M., Mente, A., Yusuf, S., 'Sodium intake and cardiovascular health', *Circ Res*, 2015, 116(6): 1046–57.

4. Rodrigues, S.L., Souza, P.R., Pimentel, E.B., et al., 'Relationship between salt consumption measured by 24-h urine collection and blood pressure in the adult population of Vitória (Brazil)', *Braz J Med Biol Res*, 2015, 48(8): 728–735.

5. Graudal, N.A., Hubeck-Graudal, T., Jurgens, G., 'Effects of low sodium diet versus high sodium diet on blood pressure, renin, aldosterone, catecholamines, cholesterol, and triglyceride', *Cochrane Database Syst Rev*, 2017, 4: CD004022.

6. He, F.J., Li, J., Macgregor, G.A., 'Effect of longer term modest salt reduction on blood pressure: Cochrane systematic review and meta-analysis of randomised trials', *BMJ*, 2013, 346: f1325.

7. Mente, A., O'Donnell, M., Rangarajan, S., 'Associations of urinary sodium excretion with cardiovascular events in individuals with and without hypertension: a pooled analysis of data from four studies', *Lancet*, 2016, 388(10043): 465–75.

8. Graudal, N.A., Hubeck-Graudal, T., Jurgens, G., 'Diet on blood pressure, renin, aldosterone, catecholamines, cholesterol, and triglyceride (Cochrane Review)', *Am J Hypertension*, 2012, 25(1): 1–15.

9. Garg, R., Williams, G.H., Hurwitz, S., et al., 'Low salt diet increases insulin resistance in healthy subjects', *Metabolism*, 2011, 60(7): 965–968.

10. DiNicolantonio, J.J., Lucan, S.C., 'The wrong white crystals: not salt but sugar as aetiological in hypertension and cardiometabolic disease', *Open Heart*, 2014, 1: e000167.

11. Yang, Q., Liu, T., Kuklina, E.V., et al., 'Sodium and potassium intake and mortality among US adults: prospective data from the Third National Health and Nutrition Examination Survey', *Arch Intern Med*, 2011, 171(13): 1183–1191.

12. Hollowell, J.G., Staehling, N.W., Hannon, W.H., 'Iodine nutrition in the United States. Trends and public health implications: iodine excretion data from National Health and Nutrition Examination Surveys I and III (1971–1974 and 1988–1994)', *J Clin Endocrinol Metab*, 1998, 83(10): 3401–8.

13. Mente, A., O'Donnell, M., Rangarajan, S., 'Associations of urinary sodium excretion with cardiovascular events'.

III. The Real Causes
Insulin Resistance

1. Kraft, J.R., *Diabetes Epidemic and You*, Trafford Publishing: Victoria, B.C., 2008.

2. Facchini, F.S., Hua, N., Abbasi, F., Reaven, G.M., 'Insulin resistance as a predictor of age-related diseases', *J Clin Endocrinol Metab*, 2001, 86(8): 3574–8.

3. Bertsch, R.A., Merchant, M.A., 'Study of the use of lipid panels as a marker of insulin resistance to determine cardiovascular risk', *Perm J*, 2015, 19(4): 4–10.

4. Weightology. https://weightology.net/insulin-an-undeserved-bad-reputation/.

Inflammation

1. Zhong, X., Guo, L., Zhang, L., et al., 'Inflammatory potential of diet and risk of cardiovascular disease or mortality: A meta-analysis', *Sci Rep*, 2017, 7(1): 6367. doi: 10.1038/s41598-017-06455-x.

2. Yang, J.S., Gerber, J.N., You, H.J., 'Association between fasting insulin and high-sensitivity C reactive protein in Korean adults', *BMJ Open Sport Exerc Med*, 2017, 3: e000236.

3. Forbes, J.D., Van Domselaar, G., Bernstein, C.N., 'The gut microbiota in immune-mediated inflammatory diseases', *Frontiers Microbiol*, 2016, 7: 1081.

4. Zhang, Y-J., Li, S., Gan, R-Y., et al., 'Impacts of gut bacteria on human health and diseases', *Int J Mol Sci*, 2015, 16(4): 7493–7519.

The Gut Microbiome

1. Lederberg, J., McCray, A.T., "Ome Sweet 'Omics—a genealogical treasury of words', *Scientist*, 2001, 15: 8.

2. Clemente, J.C., Pehrsson, E.C., Blaser, M.J., et al., 'The microbiome of uncontacted Amerindians', *Science Advances*, 2015, 1(3): e1500183; Martínez, I., Stegen, J.C., Maldonado-Gómez, M.X., et al., 'The gut microbiota of rural Papua New Guineans: composition, diversity patterns, and ecological processes', *Cell Reports*, 2015, 111(4): 527–538.

3. Mercola, J., 'The Health Benefits of Fiber', November 2013. https://articles.mercola.com/sites/articles/archive/2013/11/25/9-fiber-health-benefits.aspx.

4. Kau, A.L., Ahern, P.P., Griffin, N.W., et al., 'Human nutrition, the gut microbiome and the immune system', *Nature*, 2011, 474: 327–336.

5. Tognini, P., 'Gut microbiota: a potential regulator of neurodevelopment front cell', *Neurosci*, 2017, 11: 25.

6. Sonnenburg, E.D., Sonnenburg, J.L., 'Starving our microbial self: the deleterious consequences of a diet deficient in microbiota-accessible carbohydrates', *Cell Metabolism*, 2014, 20(5): 779–86.

7. Slingerland, A.E., Schwabkey, Z., Wiesnoski, D.H., et al., 'Clinical evidence for the microbiome in inflammatory diseases', *Front Immunol*, 2017, 8: 400.

8. Bokulich, N.A., Chung, J., Battaglia, T., 'Antibiotics, birth mode, and diet shape microbiome maturation during early life', *Sci Trans Med*, 2016, 8(343): 343ra82.

9. Fasano, A., 'Zonulin, regulation of tight junctions, and autoimmune diseases', *Ann N Y Acad Sci*, 2012, 1258(1): 25–33.

10. Rogers, G.B., Keating, D.J., Young, R.L., Wong, M-L., Licinio, J., Wesselingh, S., 'From gut dysbiosis to altered brain function and mental illness: mechanisms and pathways', *Molecular Psychiatry*, 2016, 21(6): 738–748.

11. Jiang, H., Ling, Z., Zhang, Y., 'Altered fecal microbiota composition in patients with major depressive disorder', *Brain Behav Immun*, 2015, 48: 186–194.

12. Li, Q., Han, Y., Dy, A.B.C., Hagerman, R.J., 'The gut microbiota and autism spectrum disorders', *Front Cell Neurosci*, 2017, 11: 120.

13. Backhed, F., Ding, H., Wang, T., et al., 'The gut microbiota as an environmental factor that regulates fat storage', *Proc Nat Acad Sci USA*, 2004, 101(44): 15718–15723.

14. Pollan, M., *Cooked: A Natural History of Transformation*, Penguin Books: London, 2013.

15. Sáez-Lara, M.J., Robles-Sanchez, C., Ruiz-Ojeda, F.J., et al., 'Effects of probiotics and synbiotics on obesity, insulin resistance syndrome, type 2 diabetes and non-alcoholic fatty liver disease: a review of human clinical trials', *Int J Molec Sci*, 2016, 17(6): 928.

Carbs, Fats and Proteins: Getting the Balance Right

1. Nowson, C., O'Connell, S., 'Protein requirements and recommendations for older people: A review', *Nutrients*, 2015, 7(8): 6874–6899.

2. Mitchell, C.J., Milan, A.M., Mitchell, S.M., et al., 'The effects of dietary protein intake on appendicular lean mass and muscle function in elderly men: a 10-wk randomized controlled trial', *Am J Clin Nutr*, 2017, 106(6): 1375–1383, ajcn.117.160325.

3. Berger, A., 'More than you ever wanted to know about protein & gluconeogenesis', July 2007. http://www.tuitnutrition.com/2017/07/gluconeogenesis.html.

4. Hamley, S., 'The effect of replacing saturated fat with mostly n-6 polyunsaturated fat on coronary heart disease: a meta-analysis of randomised controlled trials', *Nutr J*, 2017, 16(1): 30.

5. Santos, F.L., Esteves, S.S., da Costa Pereira, A., et al., 'Systematic review and meta-analysis of clinical trials of the effects of low carbohydrate diets on cardiovascular risk factors', *Obes Rev*, 2012, 13(11): 1048–66.

6. Simopoulos, A.P., DiNicolantonio, J.J., 'The importance of a balanced ω-6 to ω-3 ratio in the prevention and management of obesity', *Open Heart*, 2016, 3: e000385.

7. Del Gobbo, L.C., Imamura, F., Aslibekyan, S., et al., 'ω-3 Polyunsaturated fatty acid biomarkers and coronary heart disease. Pooling project of 19 cohort studies', *JAMA Intern Med*, 2016, 176(8): 1–13.

8. Menni, C., Zierer, J., Pallister, T., et al., 'Omega-3 fatty acids correlate with gut microbiome diversity and production of N-carbamylglutamate in middle aged and elderly women', *Sci Rep*, 2017, 7: 11079.

9. de Souza, R.J., Mente, A., Maroleanu, A., et al., 'Intake of saturated and trans unsaturated fatty acids and risk of all cause mortality, cardiovascular disease, and type 2 diabetes: systematic review and meta-analysis of observational studies', *BMJ*, 2015, 351: h3978.

IV. My Five Golden Rules
1. Cut Back On Sugar

1. Johnson, R.J., Segal, M.S., Sautin, Y., 'Potential role of sugar (fructose) in the epidemic of hypertension, obesity and the metabolic syndrome, diabetes, kidney disease, and cardiovascular disease', *Am J Clin Nutr*, 2007, 86(4): 899–906.

2. Australian Bureau of Statistics, 'Table 8.1 Proportion of Added Sugars(a)(b) from discretionary/non-discretionary food groups', *Australian Health Survey: Consumption of added sugars, 2011–12*.

3. Australian Bureau of Statistics, 'Consumption of sweetened beverages', 4364.0.55.007, *Australian Health Survey: Nutrition First Results – Foods and Nutrients, 2011–12*.

4. Sugar Shame. https://sugarshame2015.wordpress.com

5. Pulker, C.E., Scott, J.A., Pollard, C.M., 'Ultra-processed family foods in Australia: nutrition claims, health claims and marketing techniques', *Public Health Nutr*, 2017, 1–11.

6. Malik, V.S., Schulze, M.B., Hu, F.B., 'Intake of sugar-sweetened beverages and weight gain: a systematic review', *Am J Clin Nutr*, 2006, 84(2): 274–288; Schulze, M.B., Manson, J.E., Ludwig, D.S., et al., 'Sugar-sweetened beverages, weight gain, and incidence of type 2 diabetes in young and middle-aged women', *JAMA*, 2004, 292: 927–34.

7. Apovian, C.M., 'Sugar-sweetened soft drinks, obesity, and type 2 diabetes', *JAMA*, 2004, 292(8): 978–9.

8. InterAct Consortium, Romaguera, D., Norat, T., et al., 'Consumption of sweet beverages and type 2 diabetes incidence in European adults: results from EPIC-InterAct', *Diabetologia*, 2013, 56(7): 1520–30.

9. Yang, Q., Zhang, Z., Gregg, E.W., et al., 'Added sugar intake and cardiovascular diseases mortality among US adults', *JAMA Intern Med*, 2014, 174(4): 516–524.

10. de Koning, L., Malik, V.S., Kellogg, M.D., et al., 'Sweetened beverage consumption, incident coronary heart disease, and biomarkers of risk in men', *Circulation*, 2012, 125: 1735–41, S1.

11. Jiang, Y., Pan, Y., Rhea, P.R., et al., 'A sucrose-enriched diet promotes tumorigenesis in mammary gland in part through the 12-lipoxygenase pathway', *Cancer Res*, 2016, 76: 24–29; Mueller, N.T., Odegaard, A., Anderson, K., et al., 'Soft drink and juice consumption and risk of pancreatic cancer: The Singapore Chinese Health Study', *Cancer Epidem Biomark Prev*, 2010, 19(2): 447–455.

12. Kassaar, O., Morais, M.P., Xu, S., et al., 'Macrophage Migration Inhibitory Factor is subjected to glucose modification and oxidation in Alzheimer's Disease', *Sci Rep*, 2017, 7: 42874; Lustig, R.H., Schmidt, L.A., Brindis, C.D., 'Public health: The toxic truth about sugar', *Nature*, 2012, 487(5): 27–29.

13. Public Health Collaboration, 'Randomised controlled trials comparing low-carb

diets of less than 130g carbohydrate per day to low-fat diets of less than 35% fat of total calories'. https://phcuk.org/rcts/.

14. Mansoor, N., Vinknes, K.J., Veiered, M.B., et al., 'Effects of low-carbohydrate diets v. low-fat diets on body weight and cardiovascular risk factors: A meta-analysis of randomised controlled trials', *Br J Nutr*, 2016, 115(3): 466–479.

2. No Vegetable Oils

1. Guyenet, S., 'The American Diet', TEDxHarvard, 2012, https://www.youtube.com/watch?v=HC20OoIgG_Y.
2. Teicholz, N., *The Big Fat Surprise*.
3. Grootveld, M., Ruiz-Rodado, V., Silwood, C.I.L., 'Detection, monitoring and deleterious health effects of lipid oxidation products generated in culinary oils during thermal stressing episodes', *Inform, American Oil Chemists' Society*, 2014, 25(10): 614–624.
4. Ramsden, C.E., Zamora, D., Majchrzak-Hong, S., 'Re-evaluation of the traditional diet-heart hypothesis: analysis of recovered data from Minnesota Coronary Experiment (1968-73)', *BMJ*, 2016, 353: i1246; Ramsden, C.E., Zamora, D., Leelarthaepin, B., et al., 'Use of dietary linoleic acid for secondary prevention of coronary heart disease and death: evaluation of recovered data from the Sydney Diet Heart Study and updated meta-analysis', *BMJ*, 2013, 346: e8707.

3. Eat Real Food

1. Daley, C.A., Abbott, A., Doyle, P.S., et al., 'A review of fatty acid profiles and anti-oxidant content in grass-fed and grain-fed beef', *Nutr J*, 2010, 9: 10.
2. Fung, J., 'Meat Kills! Maybe, possibly…', *Intensive Dietary Management*. https://idmprogram.com/meat-kills-maybe-possibly/.
3. Ede, G., 'Does meat cause cancer?', *Diagnosis Diet*. http://www.diagnosisdiet.com/meat-and-cancer/.
4. Harcombe, Z., *The Obesity Epidemic: What caused it? How can we stop it?*, Columbus Publishing: Monmouthshire, 2010.
5. Virtanen, J.K., Musru, J., Tuomainen, T.P., et al., 'Egg consumption and risk of incident type 2 diabetes in men: the Kuopio Ischaemic Heart Disease Risk Factor Study', *Am J Clin Nutr*, 2015, 101(5): 1088–96.
6. Iannotti, L.L., Lutter, C.K., Stewart, C.P., et al., 'Eggs in early complementary feeding and child growth: a randomized controlled trial', *Pediatrics*, 2017, 140(1), pii: e20163459, doi: 10.1542/peds.2016-3459.
7. Gholami, F., Khoramdad, M., Esmailnasab, N., 'The effect of dairy consumption on the prevention of cardiovascular diseases: A meta-analysis of prospective studies', *J Cardiovasc Thorac Res*, 2017, 9(1): 1–11.
8. Rautiainen, S., Wang, L., Lee, I.M., et al., 'Dairy consumption in association with weight change and risk of becoming overweight or obese in middle-aged and older women: a prospective cohort study', *Am J Clin Nutr*, 2016, 103(4): 979–88.

9. Johnston, C.S., Steplewska, I., Long, C.A., et al., 'Examination of the anti-glycemic *properties of vinegar in healthy adults*', *Ann Nutr Metab*, 2010, 56(1): 74–9.

10. Damasceno, N.R., Sala Vila, A., Cofan, M., et al., 'Mediterranean diet supplemented with nuts reduces waist circumference and shifts lipoprotein subfractions to a less atherogenic pattern in subjects at high cardiovascular risk', *Atherosclerosis*, 2013, 230(2): 347–53; Garg, M.L., Blake, R.J., Wills, R.B., 'Macadamia nut consumption lowers plasma total and LDL cholesterol levels in hypercholesterolemic men', *J Nutr*, 2003, 133(4): 1060–3.

11. Ros, E., 'Health Benefits of nut consumption', *Nutrients*, 2010, 2(7): 652–682.

12. Casas, R., Sacanella, E., Urpi-Sarda, M., et al., 'The effects of the Mediterranean diet on biomarkers of vascular wall inflammation and plaque vulnerability in subjects with high risk for cardiovascular disease. A randomized trial', *PLoS One*, 2014, 9(6): e100084.

13. Joseph, M., 'A complete guide to all types of nuts', *Nutrition Advance*, 2017. http://nutritionadvance.com/types-of-nuts-complete-guide/.

14. Guasch-Ferré, M., Merino, J., Sun, Q., et al., 'Dietary polyphenols, Mediterranean diet, prediabetes, and type 2 diabetes: a narrative review of the evidence', *Oxid Med Cell Longev*, 2017, 2017: 6723931, doi: 10.1155/2017/6723931.

4. Avoid Processed Foods

1. Hu, E.A., Pan, A., Malik, V., et al., 'White rice consumption and risk of type 2 diabetes: meta-analysis and systematic review', *BMJ*, 2012, 344: e1454.

2. Perlmutter, D., *Grain Brain*, Hodder & Stoughton: London, 2014.

3. Davis, W., *Wheat Belly*, HarperCollins: London, 2015.

4. Zanini, B., Petroboni, B., Not, T., et al., 'Search for atoxic cereals: a single blind, cross-over study on the safety of a single dose of Triticum monococcum, in patients with celiac disease', *BMC Gastroenterol*, 2013, 13: 92.

5. Sofi, F., Whittaker, A., Cesani, F., et al., 'Characterization of Khorasan wheat (Kamut) and impact of a replacement diet on cardiovascular risk factors: cross-over dietary intervention study', *Eur J Clin Nutr*, 2013, 67(2): 190–5.

6. Bahrami, M., Ataie-Iafari, A., Hosseini, S., et al., 'Effects of natural honey consumption in diabetic patients: an 8-week randomized clinical trial', *Int J Food Sci Nutr*, 2009, 60(7): 618–26.

7. Kwok, C.S., Boekholdt, S.M., Lentjes, M.A.H., et al., 'Habitual chocolate consumption and risk of cardiovascular disease among healthy men and women', *Heart*, 2015, 101: 1279–1287.

5. Drink When You're Thirsty, Preferably Water

1. Feng, L., Chong, M.S., Lim, W.S., et al., 'Tea consumption reduces the incidence of neurocognitive disorders: Findings from the Singapore longitudinal aging study', *J Nutr Health Aging*, 2016, 20(10): 1002.

2. Green, R.J., Murphy, A.S., Schulz, B., et al., 'Common tea formulations modulate

in vitro digestive recovery of green tea catechins', *Mol Nutr Food Res*, 2007, 51: 1152–1162.

3. Jiang, X., Zhang, D., Juang, W., 'Coffee and caffeine intake and incidence of type 2 diabetes mellitus: a meta-analysis of prospective studies', *Eur J Nutr*, 2014, 53(1): 25–38; Ascherio, A., Zhang, S.M., Hernan, M.A., et al., 'Prospective study of caffeine consumption and risk of Parkinson's disease in men and women', *Ann Neurol*, 2001, 50(1): 56–63; Driscoll, I., Shumaker, S.A., Snively, B.M., et al., 'Relationships between caffeine intake and risk for probable dementia or global cognitive impairment: the Women's Health Initiative memory study', *J Gerontol (A)*, 2016, 71(12): 1596–1602; Schmit, S.L., Rennert, H.S., Rennert, G., et al., 'Coffee consumption and the risk of colorectal cancer', *Cancer Epidemiol Biomarkers Prev*, 2016, 25(4): 634–9; Welsh, E.J., Bara, A., Barley, E., et al., 'Caffeine for asthma', *Cochrane Database of Systematic Reviews*, 2010, 1: CD001112, doi: 10.1002/14651858.CD001112.pub2; Sang, L-X., Chang, B., Li, X-H., et al., 'Consumption of coffee associated with reduced risk of liver cancer', *BMC Gastroenterol*, 2013, 13: 34.

4. Kempf, K., Herder, C., Erlund, I., 'Effects of coffee consumption on subclinical inflammation and other risk factors for type 2 diabetes: a clinical trial', *Am J Clin Nutr*, 2010, 91(4): 950–7.

5. Hodgson, A.B., Randell, R.K., Jeukendrup, A.E., 'The metabolic and performance effects of caffeine compared to coffee during endurance exercise', *PLoS ONE*, 2013, 8(4): e59561.

6. Astorino, T.A., Roberson, D.W., 'Efficacy of acute caffeine ingestion for short-term high-intensity exercise performance: a systematic review', *J Strength Cond Res*, 2010, 24(1): 257–65.

7. 'Recipe: How to Make Bulletproof Coffee … And Make Your Morning Bulletproof', *Bulletproof*. https://blog.bulletproof.com/how-to-make-your-coffee-bulletproof-and-your-morning-too/.

8. Wikoff, D., Welsh, B.T., Henerson, R., et al., 'Systematic review of the potential adverse effects of caffeine consumption in healthy adults, pregnant women, adolescents, and children', *Food Chem Toxicol*, 2017, 109: 585–648.

9. Poole, R., Kennedy, O.J., Roderick, P., et al., 'Coffee consumption and health: umbrella review of meta-analyses of multiple health outcomes', *BMJ*, 2017, 359: j5024.

10. Hansen, A.S., Marckmann, P., Dragsted, L.O., et al., 'Effect of red wine and red grape extract on blood lipids, haemostatic factors, and other risk factors for cardiovascular disease', *Eur J Clin Nutr*, 2005, 59(3): 449–55.

11. Queipo-Ortuno, M.I., Boto-Ordonez, M., Murri, M., 'Influence of red wine polyphenols and ethanol on the gut microbiota ecology and biochemical biomarkers', *Am J Clin Nutr*, 2012, 95(6): 1323–34.

12. Australian Government, 'Nutrient Reference Values for Australia and New Zealand', 2005. https://www.nrv.gov.au/nutrients/water.

V. How to Eat Well for Life
The Trouble with Weight-loss Diets

1. Bijlefeld, M., Zoumbaris, S.K., *Encyclopedia of Diet Fads*. Greenwood Press: Westport, C.T., 2003.
2. Mann, T., Tomiyama, A.J., Westling, E., et al., 'Medicare's search for effective obesity treatments: diets are not the answer', *Am Psychol*, 2007, 62(3): 220–33.
3. Polidori, D., Sanghvi, A., Seeley, R.J., et al., 'How strongly does appetite counter weight loss? Quantification of the feedback control of human energy intake', *Obesity*, 2016, 24(11): 2289–95.
4. Zheng, M., Rangan, A., Meertens, B., et al., 'Changes in Typical Portion Sizes of Commonly Consumed Discretionary Foods among Australian Adults from 1995 to 2011–2012', *Nutrients*, 2017, 9(6), pii: E577, doi: 10.3390/nu9060577.
5. Wansink, B., Kim, J., 'Bad popcorn in big buckets: portion size can influence intake as much as taste', *J Nutr Educ Behav*, 2005, 37(5): 242–5.

Don't Blow the Food Budget

1. Lee, A.J., Kane, S., Ramsey, R., et al., 'Testing the price and affordability of healthy and current (unhealthy) diets and the potential impacts of policy change in Australia', *BMC Public Health*, 2016, 16: 315.
2. Quoted in Rachel Clemons, 'Is a healthy diet expensive?', *Choice*, 22 September 2017. www.choice.com.au/food-and-drink/diet-foods/health-and-weight-loss/articles/cost-of-healthy-food.

Fast Food Doesn't Necessarily Mean Junk Food

1. DiPatrizio, N.V., Astarita, G., Schwartz, G., et al., 'Endocannabinoid signal in the gut controls dietary fat intake', *Proc Natl Acad Sci USA*, 2011, 108(31): 12904–8.

Reading Food Labels

1. 'Style guide', Health Star Rating System, 30 June 2016. healthstarrating.gov.au/internet/healthstarrating/publishing.nsf/Content/style-guide.
2. FitzSimons, P., '"It's freaking hopeless": why the Health Star Rating System has to go', *Sydney Morning Herald*, 13 June 2017. www.smh.com.au/comment/its-freaking-hopeless-the-health-star-rating-system-has-to-go-20170611-gwp0mb.html.

Supplements

1. Pasiakos, S.M., Lieberman, H.R., McLellan, T.M., 'Effects of protein supplements on muscle damage, soreness and recovery of muscle function and physical performance: a systematic review', *Sports Med*, 2014, 44(5): 655–70.
2. Geleijnse, J.M., Vermeer, C., Grobbea, D.E., et al., 'Dietary intake of menaquinone is associated with a reduced risk of coronary heart disease: the Rotterdam Study',

J Nutr, 2004, 134(11): 3100–5; Nimptsch, K., Rohrmann, S., Kaaks, R., et al., 'Dietary vitamin K intake in relation to cancer incidence and mortality: results from the Heidelberg cohort of the European Prospective Investigation into Cancer and Nutrition (EPIC-Heidelberg)', *Am J Clin Nutr*, 2010, 91(5): 1348–58.

3. Cockayne, S., Adamson, J., Lanham-New, S., et al., 'Vitamin K and the prevention of fractures: systematic review and meta-analysis of randomized controlled trials', *Arch Intern Med*, 2006, 166: 1256–61.

4. US Preventive Services Task Force, 'Vitamin D and Calcium to Prevent Fractures: Preventive Medication'. https://www.uspreventiveservicestaskforce.org/Page/Document/final-evidence-summary52/vitamin-d-and-calcium-to-prevent-fractures-preventive-medication.

5. Bolland, M.J., Avenell, A., Baron, J.A.G., et al., 'Effect of calcium supplements on risk of myocardial infarction and cardiovascular events: meta-analysis', *BMJ*, 2010, 341: c3691.

6. Rizos, E.C., Ntzani, E.E., Bika, E., et al., 'Association between omega-3 fatty acid supplementation and risk of major cardiovascular disease events: a systematic review and meta-analysis', *JAMA*, 2012, 308(10): 1024–33.

7. Erkkila, A.T., Lichtenstein, A.H., Mozaffarian, D., et al., 'Fish intake is associated with a reduced progression of coronary artery atherosclerosis in postmenopausal women with coronary artery disease', *Am J Clin Nutr*, 2004, 80(3): 626–632.

8. Menon, V.P., Sudheer, A.R., 'Antioxidant and anti-inflammatory properties of curcumin', *Adv Exp Med Biol*, 2007, 595: 105–25.

9. Shoba, G., Joy, D., Joseph, T., et al., 'Influence of piperine on the pharmacokinetics of curcumin in animals and human volunteers', *Planta Med*, 1998, 64(4): 353–6.

Sweeteners

1. Mordor Intelligence, 'Food Sweetener Market – Growth, Trends, Forecast for the period (2017–2022)', November 2017. https://www.mordorintelligence.com/industry-reports/global-food-sweetener-market-industry.

2. PubMed Health, 'Reported link between diet drinks and dementia and stroke is weak', April 2017. https://www.ncbi.nlm.nih.gov/pubmedhealth/behindtheheadlines/news/2017-04-21-reported-link-between-diet-drinks-and-dementia-and-stroke-is-weak/.

3. Papier, K., D'Este, C., Bain, C., et al., 'Consumption of sugar-sweetened beverages and type 2 diabetes incidence in Thai adults: results from an 8-year prospective study', *Nutr Diabetes*, 2017, 7: e283.

4. Fagherazzi, G., Vilier, A., Saes Sartorelli, D., et al., 'Consumption of artificially and sugar-sweetened beverages and incident type 2 diabetes in the Etude Epidémiologique auprès des femmes de la Mutuelle Générale de l'Education Nationale–European Prospective Investigation into Cancer and Nutrition cohort', *Am J Clin Nutr*, 2013, 97(3): 517–23.

5. Suez, J., Korem, T., Zeevi, D., et al., 'Artificial sweeteners induce glucose intolerance by altering the gut microbiota', *Nature*, 2014, 514: 181–186.

6. Nettleton, J.A., Lutsey, P.L., Wang, Y., et al., 'Diet soda intake and risk of incident metabolic syndrome and type 2 diabetes in the multi-ethnic study of athero-sclerosis (MESA)', *Diabetes Care*, 2009, 32(4): 688–694.

7. Azad, M.B., Abou-Setta, A.M., Chauhan, B.F., et al., 'Nonnutritive sweeteners and cardiometabolic health: a systematic review and meta-analysis of randomized controlled trials and prospective cohort studies', *CMAJ*, 2017, 189(28): E929–E939.

8. Suez, J., Korem, T., Zeevi, D., et al., 'Artificial sweeteners induce glucose intolerance by altering the gut microbiota', *Nature*, 2014, 514: 181–6.

9. Nayak, P.A., Nayak, U.A., Khandelwal, V., 'The effect of xylitol on dental caries and oral flora', *Clin Cosmet Investig Dent*, 2014, 6: 89–94.

10. Mattila, P.T., Svanberg, M.J., Knuuttila, M.L., 'Increased bone volume and bone mineral content in xylitol-fed aged rats', *Gerontology*, 2001, 47(6): 300–5.

11. Aune, D., 'Soft drinks, aspartame, and the risk of cancer and cardiovascular disease', *Am J Clin Nutr*, 2012, 96(6): 1249–51.

12. Schernhammer, E.S., Bertrand, K.A., Birmann, B.M., et al., 'Consumption of artificial sweetener- and sugar-containing soda and risk of lymphoma and leukemia in men and women', *Am J Clin Nutr*, 2012, 96(6): 1419–28.

13. Soffritti, M., Padovani, M., Tibaldi, E., et al., 'Sucralose administered in feed, beginning prenatally through lifespan, induces hematopoietic neoplasias in male Swiss mice', *Int J Occup Environ Health*, 2016, 22(1): 7–17.

14. Sharma, N., Mogra, N.R., Upadhyay, B., 'Effect of Stevia extract intervention on lipid profile', *Ethno-Med*, 2009, 3(2): 137–140.

15. Bahrami, M., Ataie-Iafari, A., Hoseini, S., et al., 'Effects of natural honey consumption in diabetic patients: an 8-week randomized clinical trial', *Int J food Sci Nutr*, 2009, 60(7): 618–626.

16. Al-Waili, N.S., 'Natural honey lowers plasma glucose, C-reactive protein, homocysteine, and blood lipids in healthy, diabetic, and hyperlipidemic subjects: comparison with dextrose and sucrose', *J Med Food*, 2004, 7(1): 100–7.

Gluten and other allergies

1. Hadjivassiliou, M., Sanders, D.S., Grunewald, R.A., et al., 'Gluten sensitivity: from gut to brain', *Lancet Neurol*, 2010, 9(3): 318–30.

2. Skodie, G.I., Sarna, V.K., Minelle, I.H., et al., 'Fructan, rather than gluten, induces symptoms in patients with self-reported non-celiac gluten sensitivity', *Gastroenterology*, 2017, pii: S0016-5085(17): 36302–3, doi: http://dx.doi.org/10.1053/j.gastro.2017.10.040.

3. Kristiansson, G., Venge, P., Hallgrens, R., 'Mucosal reactivity to cow's milk protein in coeliac disease', *Clin Exp Immunol*, 2007, 147(3): 449–455.

4. Prescott. S, Pawankar, R., Allen, K.J., et al., 'A global survey of changing patterns of food allergy burden in children', *World Allergy Organ J*, 2013, 6(1): 21.

5. Abrahamsson, T.R., Jakobsson, H.E., Andersson, A.F., et al., 'Low diversity of the gut microbiota in infants with atopic eczema', *J Allergy Clin Immunol*, 2012, 129(2): 434–40.

6. Metsala, J., Lundqvist, A., Virta, L.J., et al., 'Mother's and offspring's use of antibiotics and infant allergy to cow's milk', *Epidemiology*, 2013, 24(2): 303–9; Yang, S-N., Hsieh, C-C., Kuo H-F., et al., 'The effects of environmental toxins on allergic inflammation', *Allergy Asthma Immunol Res*, 2014, 6(6): 478–484; Myles, I.A., 'Fast food fever: reviewing the impacts of the Western diet on immunity', *Nutr J*, 2014, 13: 61; Renz-Polster, H., David, M.R., Buist, A.S., 'Caesarean section delivery and the risk of allergic disorders in childhood', *Clin Exp Allergy*, 2005, 35(11): 1466–72; Guaraldi, F., Salvatori, G., 'Effect of breast and formula feeding on gut microbiota shaping in newborns', *Front Cell Infect Microbiol*, 2012, 2: 94; Hanski, I., von Hertzen, L., Fyhrquist, N., et al., 'Environmental biodiversity, human microbiota, and allergy are interrelated', *Proc Natl Acad Sci USA*, 2012, 109(21): 8334–9.

7. Castellazzi, A.M., Valsecchi, C., Caimmi, S., et al., 'Probiotics and food allergy', *Ital J Pediatr*, 2013, 39: 47.

Vegetarian and Vegan Diets

1. Craig, W.J., 'Nutrition concerns and health effects of vegetarian diets', *Nutr Clin Pract*, 2010, 25(6): 613–20.

2. Rosell, M.S., Lloyd-Wright, Z., Appleby, P.N., et al., 'Long-chain n-3 polyunsaturated fatty acids in plasma in British meat-eating, vegetarian, and vegan men', *Am J Clin Nutr*, 2005, 82(2): 327–34.

The Ketogenic Diet

1. Joseph, M., *The Ketogenic Diet: An Ultimate Guide to Keto*, February 2017. http://nutritionadvance.com/ketogenic-diet-ultimate-guide-to-keto/.

Female-specific Issues

1. McGrice, M., Porter, J., 'The effect of low carbohydrate diets on fertility hormones and outcomes in overweight and obese women: a systematic review', *Nutrients*, 2017, 9(3): 204.

2. Donnelly, L., 'Go "low carb" to increase fertility chances by five times, experts say', *The Telegraph*, 5 July 2017. http://www.telegraph.co.uk/news/2017/07/05/go-low-carb-increase-fertility-chances-five-times-experts-say/.

3. Joham, A.E., Ranasinha, S., Zoungas, S., et al., 'Gestational diabetes and type 2 diabetes in reproductive-aged women with polycystic ovary syndrome', *J Clin Endocrinol Metab*, 2014, 99(3): E447–52.

4. Way, K.L., Hackett, D.A., Baker, M.K., et al., 'The effect of regular exercise on insulin sensitivity in type 2 diabetes mellitus: a systematic review and meta-analysis', *Diabetes Metab J*, 2016, 40(4): 253–271.

5. Ding, C., Parameswaran, V., Udavan, R., et al., 'Circulating levels of inflammatory markers predict change in bone mineral density and resorption in older adults: a longitudinal study', *J Clin Endocrinol Metab*, 2008, 93(5): 1952–8.

6. Orchard, T., Yildiz, V., Steck, S.E., 'Dietary inflammatory index, bone mineral density, and risk of fracture in postmenopausal women: results from the Women's Health Initiative', *J Bone Miner Res*, 2017, 32(5): 1136–1146.

Feeding Kids

1. Leung, J., Funder, J. 'Obesity: A national epidemic and its impact on Australia', *Obesity Australia*, 2014. https://static1.squarespace.com/static/57e9ebb16a4963ef7 adfafdb/t/580ec0679de4bb7cf16ffb9a/1477361771570/NTTW%2BReport.pdf.

2. Vanderhout, S.M., Birken, C.S., Parkin, P.C., et al., 'Relation between milk-fat percentage, vitamin D, and BMI z score in early childhood', *Am J Clin Nutr*, 2016, 104(6): 1657–1664.

Diet and Sports Performance

1. Dickinson, M., 'My sporting body, by Chris Froome', *The Times*, 16 September 2017. www.thetimes.co.uk/article/my-sporting-body-by-chris-froome-fbcfpk8cp.

VI. The S-entials of Healthy Living
Avoid Sedentary Behaviour: Exercise

1. Koolhaas, C.M., Dhana, K., Schoufour, J.D., et al., 'Impact of physical activity on the association of overweight and obesity with cardiovascular disease: The Rotterdam Study', *Eur J Prev Cardiol*, 2017, 24(9): 934–941.

2. Meyer, J.D., Koltyn, K.F., Stegner, A.J., et al., 'Influence of exercise intensity for improving depressed mood in depression: a dose-response study', *Behav Ther*, 2016, 47(4): 527–37; Pedrinolla, A., Schena, F., Venturelli, M., et al., 'Resilience to Alzheimer's disease: the role of physical activity', *Curr Alzheimer Res*, 2017.

3. Cormie, P., Zopf, E.M., Zhang, X., et al., 'The impact of exercise on cancer mortality, recurrence, and treatment-related adverse effects', *Epidemiol Rev*, 2017, 39(1): 71–92.

4. Warburton, D.E.R, Nicol, C.W., Bredin, S.S.D., 'Health benefits of physical activity: the evidence', *CMAJ*, 2006, 174(6): 801–809.

5. Gebel. K., Ding. D., Chey, T., et al., 'Effect of moderate to vigorous physical activity on all-cause mortality in middle-aged and older Australians', *JAMA Intern Med*, 2015, 175: 970–7.

6. Freedhoff, Y., '"Constrained energy expenditures" and not outrunning our forks', *Weight Matters*, 1 February 2016. www.weightymatters.ca/2016/02/constrained-energy-expenditures-and-not.html.

7. Malhotra, A., Noakes, T., Phinney, S., 'It is time to bust the myth of physical inactivity and obesity: you cannot outrun a bad diet', *Br J Sports Med*, 2015, 49(15): 967–8.

8. Kerns, J.C., Guo, J., Fothergill, E., et al., 'Increased physical activity associated with less weight regain six years after "the biggest loser" competition', *Obesity*, 2017, 25(11): 1838–1843.

9. Australian Bureau of Statistics, 'Table 8.3', *National Health Survey: First Results, 2014–15*.

10. Heart Foundation. https://www.heartfoundation.org.au/active-living/get-active.

11. Thornton, J.S., Frémont, P., Khan, K., et al., 'Physical activity prescription: A critical opportunity to address modifiable risk factor for the prevention and management of chronic disease: a position statement by the Canadian Academy of Sport and Exercise Medicine', *Br J Sports Med*, 2016, 50(18): 1109–14.

12. Diaz, K.M., Howard, V.J., Hutt, B., et al., 'Patterns of sedentary behavior and mortality in U.S. middle-aged and older adults: a national cohort study', *Ann Intern Med*, 2017, 167(7): 465–475; van der Ploeg, H.P., Chey, T., Korda, R.J., et al., 'Sitting time and all-cause mortality risk in 222,497 Australian adults', *Arch Intern Med*, 2012, 172(6): 494–500.

13. Costigan, S.A., Eather, N., Plotnikoff, R.C., et al., 'High-intensity interval training for improving health-related fitness in adolescents: a systematic review and meta-analysis', *Br J Sports Med*, 2015, 49(19): 1253–61; Batacan, R.B., Duncan, M.J., Dalbo, V.J., et al., 'Effects of high-intensity interval training on cardiometabolic health: a systematic review and meta-analysis of intervention studies', *Br J Sports Med*, 2017, 51: 494–503.

14. Nieuwoudt, S., Fealy, C.E., Foucher, J.A., et al., 'Functional high intensity training improves pancreatic β-cell function in adults with type 2 diabetes', *Am J Physiol Endocrinol Metab*, 2017, 313(3): E314–E320. doi: 10.1152/ajpendo.00407.2016.

15. Phillips, B.E., Kelly, B.M., Lilia, M., 'A practical and time-efficient high-intensity interval training program modifies cardio-metabolic risk factors in adults with risk factors for type ii diabetes', *Front Endocrinol*, 2017, 8: 229.

16. Rantanen, T., Harris, T., Leveille, S.G., et al., 'Muscle strength and body mass index as long-term predictors of mortality in initially healthy men', *J Gerontol A*, 2000, 55(3): M168–M173.

17. Winett, R.A., Carpinelli, R.N., 'Potential health-related benefits of resistance training', *Prev Med*, 2001, 33(5): 503–13.

18. Behm, D.G., Blazevich, A.J., Kay, A.D., 'Acute effects of muscle stretching on physical performance, range of motion, and injury incidence in healthy active individuals: a systematic review', *Appl Physiol Nutr Metab*, 2016, 41(1): 1–11.

Achieve More Good-Quality Sleep

1. Sleep Health Foundation, *Asleep on the Job: Costs of inadequate sleep in Australia*, 2017. https://www.sleephealthfoundation.org.au/files/Asleep_on_the_job/Asleep_on_the_Job_SHF_report-WEB_small.pdf.

2. Cappuccio, F.P., Taggart, F.M., Kandala, N.B., et al., 'Meta-analysis of short sleep duration and obesity in children and adults', *Sleep*, 2008, 31: 619–626; Sperry, S.D., Scully, I.D., Gramzow, R.H., et al., 'Sleep duration and waist circumference in adults: a meta-analysis', *Sleep*, 2015, 38: 1269–1276.

3. Carter, P.J., Taylor, B.J., Williams, S.M., et al., 'Longitudinal analysis of sleep in relation to BMI and body fat in children: the FLAME study', *BMJ*, 2011, 342: d2712.

4. Chahal, H., Fung, C., Kuhle, S., 'Availability and night-time use of electronic entertainment and communication devices are associated with short sleep duration and obesity among Canadian children', *Podiatry Obes*, 2013, 8(1): 42–51.

5. Taheri, S., Lin, L., Austin, D., et al., 'Short sleep duration is associated with reduced leptin, elevated ghrelin, and increased body mass index', *PLoS Med*, 2004,1(3): e62.

6. Al Khatib, H.K., Harding, S.V., Darzi, J., et al., 'The effects of partial sleep deprivation on energy balance: a systematic review and meta-analysis', *Eur J Clin Nutr*, 2017, 71: 614–624.

7. Mesarwi, O., Polak, J., Jun, J., 'Sleep disorders and the development of insulin resistance and obesity', *Endocrinol Metab Clin North Am*, 2013, 42(3): 617–34.

8. Morselli, L., Leproult, R., Balbo, M., et al., 'Role of sleep deprivation in the regulation of glucose metabolism and appetite', *Best Pract Res Clin Endocrinol Metab*, 2010, 24(5): 687–702.

9. AlDabal, L., BaHammam, A.S., 'Metabolic, endocrine, and immune consequences of sleep deprivation', *Open Respir Med J*, 2011, 5: 31–43.

10. Esther Donga, E., van Dijk, M., van Dijk, J.G., et al., 'A single night of partial sleep deprivation induces insulin resistance in multiple metabolic pathways in healthy subjects', *J Clin Endocrinol Metab*, 2010, 95(6): 2963–8.

11. Alhola, P., Polo-Kantola, P., 'Sleep deprivation: Impact on cognitive performance', *Neuropsychiatr Dis Treat*, 2007, 3(5): 553–567.

12. Spira, A.P., Gamaldo, A.A., An, Y., et al., 'Self-reported sleep and β-amyloid deposition in community-dwelling adults', *JAMA Neurol*, 2013, 70(12): 1537–43.

13. European Society of Cardiology, 'Poor sleep associated with increased risk of heart attack, stroke: Poor sleep should be considered a risk factor for cardiovascular disease along with smoking, lack of exercise and poor diet', *ScienceDaily*, 15 June 2015. www.sciencedaily.com/releases/2015/06/150615094255.htm.

14. Mullington, J.M., Simpson, N.S., Meier-Ewert, H.K., et al., 'Sleep Loss and Inflammation', *Best Pract Res Clin Endocrinol Metab*, 2010, 24(5): 775–784.

15. Ashwin, N., Ananthakrishnan, A.N., Khalili, H., Konijeti, G.G., et al., 'Sleep duration affects risk for ulcerative colitis: a prospective cohort study', *Clin Gastroenterol Hepatol*, 2014, 12(11): 1879–86.

16. Carey, B., 'Sleep Therapy Seen as an Aid for Depression', *New York Times*, 18 November 2013. http://www.nytimes.com/2013/11/19/health/treating-insomnia-to-heal-depression.html?pagewanted=1&_r=1&nl=todaysheadlines&emc=edit_th_20131119&&pagewanted=all.

17. Bernert, R.A., Turvey, C.L., Conwell, Y., et al., 'Association of poor subjective sleep quality with risk for death by suicide during a 10-year period: a longitudinal, population-based study of late life', *JAMA Psychiatry*, 2014, 71(10): 1129–37.

18. Smedje, H., Broman, J.E. and Hetta, J., 'Associations between disturbed sleep and behavioural difficulties in 635 children aged six to eight years: a study based on parents' perceptions', *Eur Child Adol Psych*, 2001, 10: 1.

19. Sigurdardottir, L.G., Valdimarsdottir, U.A., Mucci, L.A., 'Sleep disruption among older men and risk of prostate cancer', *Cancer Epidemiol Biomarkers Prev*, 2013, 22(5): 872–9.

20. Schernhammer, E.S., Laden, F., Speizer, F.E., 'Rotating night shifts and risk of breast cancer in women participating in the nurses' health study', *J Natl Cancer Inst*, 2001, 93(20): 1563–8.

21. Milewski, M.D., Skaggs, D.L., Bishop, G.A., 'Chronic lack of sleep is associated with increased sports injuries in adolescent athletes', *J Pediatr Orthop*, 2014, 34(2): 129–33.

22. Luke, A., Lazaro, R.M., Bergeron, M.F., et al., 'Sports-related injuries in youth athletes: is overscheduling a risk factor?', *Clin J Sport Med*, 2011, 21(4): 307–14.

23. Lee, W., Nagubadi, S., Kryger, M.H., et al., 'Epidemiology of obstructive sleep apnea: a population-based perspective', *Expert Rev Respir Med*, 2008, 2(3): 349–364.

24. Romero-Corral, A., Caples, S.M., Lopez-Jimenez, F., et al., 'Interactions between obesity and obstructive sleep apnea: implications for treatment', *Chest*, 2010, 137(3): 711–719.

25. Snore Australia, 'Obstructive Sleep Apnoea'. http://www.snoreaustralia.com.au/obstructive-sleep-apnoea.php.

26. NODSS, 'Sleep Apnoea'. http://www.nodss.org.au/sleep_apnoeas.html.

Reduce Stress

1. Vogelzangs, N., Beekman, A.T.F, Milaneschi, Y., et al., 'Urinary cortisol and six-year risk of all-cause and cardiovascular mortality', *J Clin Endocrinol Metab*, 2010, 95(11): 4959–4964.

2. Hertig, V.L., Cain, K.C., Jarrett, M.E., 'Daily stress and gastrointestinal symptoms in women with irritable bowel syndrome', *Nurs Res*, 2007, 56(6): 399–406.

3. Jackson, S.E., Kirschbaum, C., Steptoe, A., 'Hair cortisol and adiposity in a population-based sample of 2,527 men and women aged 54 to 87 years', *Obesity*, 2017, 25(3): 539–544.

4. Qu, S., Olafsund, S.M., Meza-Zepeda, L.A., et al., 'Rapid gene expression changes in peripheral blood lymphocytes upon practice of a comprehensive yoga program', *PLoS One*, 2013, 8(4): e61910.

5. Benson, H., *The Relaxation Response*, New York: HarperTorch, 2000.

6. Goleman, D., Davidson, R.J., *Altered Traits*, New York: Penguin Random House, 2017.

Get Moderate Sun Exposure

1. Elwood, J.M., Jopson, J., 'Melanoma and sun exposure: an overview of published studies', *Int J Cancer*, 1997, 73(2): 198–203.

2. Lou, Y-R., Peng, Q-Y., Li, T., et al., 'Effects of high-fat diets rich in either omega-3 or omega-6 fatty acids on UVB-induced skin carcinogenesis in SKH-1 mice', *Carcinogenesis*, 2011, 32(7): 1078–1084.

3. Juzeniene, A., Moan, J., 'Beneficial effects of UV radiation other than via vitamin D production', *Dermato-endocrinology*, 2012, 4(2): 109–117.

4. O'Gorman, C., Lucas, R., Taylor, B., 'Environmental risk factors for multiple sclerosis: a review with a focus on molecular mechanisms', *Int J Mol Sci*, 2012, 13(9): 11718–11752.

5. Xiong, S., Sankaridurg, P., Naduvilath, T., et al., 'Time spent in outdoor activities in relation to myopia prevention and control: a meta-analysis and systematic review', *Acta Ophthalmol*, 2007, 95: 551–566.

6. Gandini, S., Autier, P., Bonici, M., 'Reviews on sun exposure and artificial light and melanoma', *Prog Biophys Mol Biol*, 2011, 107(3): 362–6.

7. Christodolou, S., Goulia, T., Verevridis, A., et al., 'Vitamin D and bone disease', *Biomed Res Int*, 2013, 2013, 396541, doi: 10.1155/2013/396541; Chowdhury, R., Kunutsor, S., Vitezova, A., et al., 'Vitamin D and risk of cause soecific death: systematic review and meta-analysis of observational cohort and randomized intervention studies', *BMJ*, 2014, 348: g1903; Girgis, C.M., Clifton-Bligh, R.J., et al., 'Effects of vitamin D in skeletal muscle: falls, strength, athletic performance and insulin sensitivity', *Clin Endocrinol (Oxf)*, 2014, 80(2): 169–81; Rebel, H., der Spek, C.D., Salvatori, D., et al., 'UV exposure inhibits intestinal tumor growth and progression to malignancy in intestine-specific Apc mutant mice kept on low vitamin D diet', *Int J Cancer*, 2014, 136: 271–7; Mohr, S.B., Gorham, E.D., Kim, J., et al., 'Meta-analysis of vitamin D sufficiency for improving survival of patients with breast cancer', *Anticancer Res*, 2014, 34: 1163–6; Millen, A.E., Meyers, K.J., Liu, Z., et al., 'Association between vitamin D status and age-related macular degeneration by genetic risk', *JAMA Ophthalmol*, 2015, 133: 1171–9; Svenningsson, P., Chergui, K., Rachleff, I., et al., 'Alterations in 5-HT1B receptor function by p11 in depression-like states', *Science*, 2006, 311: 77–80; Littlejohns, T.J., Henley, W.E., Lang, I.A., et al., 'Vitamin D the risk of dementia and Alzheimer disease', *Neurology*, 2014, 83: 920–8; Mirhosseini, N., Vatanparat, H., Mazidi, M., et al., 'The effect of improved serum 25-hydroxyvitamin d status on glycemic control in diabetic patients: a meta-analysis', *J Clin Endocrinol Metab*, 2017, 102: 3097–3110; Mitri, J., Muraru, M.D., Pittas, A.G., 'Vitamin D and type 2 diabetes: a systematic review', *Eur J Clin Nutr*, 2011, 65: 1005–15; Rimmelzwaan, L.M., van Schoor, N.M., Lips, P., et al., 'Systematic review of the relationship between vitamin D and Parkinsons disease', *J Parkinsons Dis*, 2016, 6(1): 29–37; McDonnell, S., Baggerly, K., Baggerly, C., et al., 'Maternal 25(OH)D

concentrations >40ng/ml associated with 60% lower preterm birth risk among general obstetrical patients at an urban medical center', *PLoS One*, 2017, 12(7): e0180483.

8. Martineau, A.R., Jolliffe, D.A., Hooper, R.L., et al., 'Vitamin D supplementation to prevent acute respiratory tract infections: systematic review and meta-analysis of individual participant data', *BMJ*, 2017, 356: i6583.

9. Lindqvist, P.G., Epstein, E., Landin-Olsson, M., et al., 'Avoidance of sun exposure is a risk factor for all-cause mortality: results from the Melanoma in Southern Sweden cohort', *J Intern Med*, 2014, 276(1): 77–86.

10. Dobnig, H., Pilz, S., Scharnagl, H., et al., 'Independent association of low serum 25-hydroxyvitamin D and 1,25-dihydroxyvitamin D levels with all-cause and cardiovascular mortality', *Arch Intern Med*, 2008, 168(12): 1340–1349.

Don't Smoke

1. GBD 2015 Tobacco Collaborators, 'Smoking prevalence and attributable disease burden in 195 countries and territories, 1990-2015: a systematic analysis from the Global Burden of Disease Study 2015', *Lancet,* 2017, 389(10082): 1885–1906.

2. U.S. Department of Health and Human Services, *The Health Consequences of Smoking: 50 Years of Progress. A Report of the Surgeon General*, Atlanta, GA: U.S. Department of Health and Human Services, Centers for Disease Control and Prevention, National Center for Chronic Disease Prevention and Health Promotion, Office on Smoking and Health, 2014. https://www.cdc.gov/tobacco/data_statistics/sgr/50th-anniversary/index.htm.

3. U.S. Department of Health and Human Services, *Health Effects of Cigarette Smoking*, Atlanta, GA: U.S. Department of Health and Human Services, Centers for Disease Control and Prevention, National Center for Chronic Disease Prevention and Health Promotion, Office on Smoking and Health. https://www.cdc.gov/tobacco/data_statistics/fact_sheets/health_effects/effects_cig_smoking/index.htm.

4. Greenhalgh, E.M., Stillman, S., Ford, C., '7.2 Quitting activity' in Scollo, M.M. and Winstanley, M.H. (ed.), *Tobacco in Australia: Facts and issues.* Melbourne: Cancer Council Victoria, 2016. http://www.tobaccoinaustralia.org.au/chapter-7-cessation/7-1-quitting-activity.

5. Help with Smoking, 'Ways to Give Up Smoking'. https://www.helpwithsmoking.com/ways-to-quit-smoking.php.

6. Public Health England, *E-cigarettes: an evidence update*, 2015. https://www.gov.uk/government/publications/e-cigarettes-an-evidence-update.

VII. Tackling the Modern Epidemics
1. Obesity

1. Malhotra, A., Noakes, T., Phinney, S., 'It is time to bust the myth', *Br J Sports Med*.

2. Medibank, *Medibank Better Health Index*, 2016. https://www.medibank.com.au/

livebetter/the-first-medibank-better-health-index-reveals-the-state-of-australias-health/.

2. Type 2 Diabetes

1. Feinman, R.D., Pogozelski, W.K., Astrup, A., et al., 'Dietary carbohydrate restriction as the first approach in diabetes management: critical review and evidence base', *Nutrition*, 2015, 31(1): 1–13.
2. McKenzie, A.L., Hallberg, S.J., Creighton, B.C., et al., 'A novel intervention including individualized nutritional recommendations reduces hemoglobin a1c level, medication use, and weight in type 2 diabetes', *JMIR Diabetes*, 2017, 2(1): e5.

3. Fatty Liver

1. DiNicolantonio, J.J., Subramonian, A.M., O'Keefe, J.H., 'Added fructose as a principal driver of non-alcoholic fatty liver disease: a public health crisis', *Open Heart*, 2017, 4: e000631, doi:10.1136/openhrt-2017-000631.

4. Tooth Decay

1. Moynihan, P.J., Kelly, S.A., 'Effect on caries of restricting sugars intake: systematic review to inform WHO guidelines', *J Dent Res*, 2014, 93(1): 8–18; Hujoel, P., 'Dietary carbohydrates and dental-systemic diseases', *J Dent Res*, 2009, 88(6): 490–502; Scientific Advisory Committee on Nutrition, *Draft Carbohydrates and Health Report*, 2014, 89–90 and 95–96. https://www.gov.uk/government/groups/scientific-advisory-committee-on-nutrition.
2. Sugarfree Smiles. sugarfreesmiles.com
3. Moynihan, P.J., 'The role of diet and nutrition in the etiology and prevention of oral diseases', *Bull WHO*, 2005, 83: 694–9.
4. Oral Health CRC, *Briefing Paper: The potential of sugar-free beverages, sugar-free confectionery and sports drinks to cause dental erosion*, 2015. https://oralhealthcrc.org.au/sites/default/files/Dental%20Erosion%20Briefing%20Paper_FINAL2015.pdf.
5. Woelber, J.P., Bremer, K., Vach, K., 'An oral health optimized diet can reduce gingival and periodontal inflammation in humans – a randomized controlled pilot study', *BMC Oral Health*, 2017, 17: 28.

5. Cardiovascular Disease

1. Sidney, S., Quesenberry, C.P., Jaffe, M.G. et al., 'Recent trends in cardiovascular mortality in the United States and public health goals', *JAMA Cardiol*, 2016, 1(5): 594–599.
2. Farrell, S.W., Finley, C.E., Barlow, C.E., et al., 'Moderate to high levels of cardiorespiratory fitness attenuate the effects of triglyceride to high-density lipoprotein cholesterol ratio on coronary heart disease mortality in men', *Mayo Clinic Proceedings*, 2017, doi: 10.1016/j.mayocp.2017.08.015.
3. Taylor, F., Huffman, M.D., Macedo, A.F. et al., 'Statins for the primary prevention

of cardiovascular disease', *Cochrane Database of Systematic Reviews*, 2013, 1: CD004816.

4. Han, B.H., Sutin, D., Williamson, J.D., et al., 'Effect of statin treatment vs usual care on primary cardiovascular prevention among older adults. The ALLHAT-LLT randomized clinical trial', *JAMA Intern Me*, 2017, 177(7): 955–965.

5. One example of an online triglycerides to HDL calculator can be found at: http://www.hughcalc.org/chol-si.php.

6. Iwani, N.A.K.Z., Jalaludin, M.Y., Zin, R.M.W.M., et al., 'Triglyceride to HDL-C ratio is associated with insulin resistance in overweight and obese children', *Sci Rep*, 2017, 7: 40055.

7. Gaziano, J.M., Hennekens, C.H., O'Donnell, C.J., et al., 'Fasting triglycerides, high-density lipoprotein, and risk of myocardial infarction', *Circulation*, 1997, 96: 2520–2525.

8. Sharma, R.K., Sharma, R.K., Voelker, D.J., et al., 'Cardiac risk stratification: Role of the coronary calcium score', *Vasc Health Risk Manag*, 2010, 6: 603–611; Jain, A., McClelland, J.A., Polak, J.F., et al., 'Cardiovascular Imaging for assessing cardiovascular risk in asymptomatic men versus women. The Multi-Ethnic Study of Atherosclerosis (MESA)', *Circ Cardiovasc Imaging*, 2010, 4(1): 8–15.

6. Chronic Diseases

1. De la Monte, S.M., 'Type 3 diabetes is sporadic Alzheimer's disease: Mini-review', *Eur Neuropsychopharmacol*, 2014, 24(12): 1954–1960.

2. Blázquez, E., Velázquez, E., Hurtado-Carneiro, V., et al., 'Insulin in the brain: its pathophysiological implications for states related with central insulin resistance, type 2 diabetes and Alzheimer's Disease', *Front Endocrinol*, 2014, 5: 161.

3. Kassaar, O., Pereira Morais, M., Xu, S., et al., 'Macrophage Migration Inhibitory Factor is subjected to glucose modification and oxidation in Alzheimer's Disease', *Sci Rep*, 2017, 7: 42874.

4. Pase, M.P., Himali, J.J., Jacques, P.F., 'Sugary beverage intake and preclinical Alzheimer's disease in the community', *Alzheimers Dement*, 2017, 13(9): 955–964.

5. Swerdlow, R., Sullivan, D., Taylor, M., 'The ketogenic diet retention and feasibility trial (KDRAFT)', *Alzheimer's Association International conference*, London UK, July 2017.

6. Krokorian, R., Shidler, M.D., Dangelo, K., et al., 'Dietary ketosis enhances memory in mild cognitive impairment', *Neurobiol Aging*, 2012, 33(2): 425, e19-27.

7. Warburg, O., 'On the origin of cancer cells', *Science*, 1956, 123(3191): 309–14.

8. Allen, B.G., Bhatia, S.K., Anderson, C.M., et al., 'Ketogenic diets as an adjuvant cancer therapy: History and potential mechanism', *Redox Biology*, 2014, 2: 963–970.

9. Zhou, W., Mukherjee, P., Kiebish, M.A., et al., 'The calorically restricted ketogenic diet, an effective alternative therapy for malignant brain cancer', *Nutr Metab*, 2007, 4: 5.

10. Schwartz, K., Chang, H.T., Nikolai, M., et al., 'Treatment of glioma patients with ketogenic diets: report of two cases treated with an IRB-approved energy-restricted ketogenic diet protocol and review of the literature', *Cancer Metab*, 2015, 3: 3.

11. Brandhorst, S., Longo, V.D., 'Fasting and Caloric Restriction in Cancer Prevention and Treatment', *Recent Results Cancer Res*, 2016, 207: 241–66.

12. Wheless, J.W., 'History of the ketogenic diet', *Epilepsia*, 2008, 49 Suppl 8: 3–5.

13. Hartman, A.L., Gasior, M., Vining, E.P.G, et al., 'The neuropharmacology of the ketogenic diet', *Pediatr neurol*, 2007, 36(5): 281–292.

14. The Charlie Foundation for Ketogenic Therapies. www.charliefoundation.org.

15. Wahls, T., 'Minding your mitochondria', TEDx, terrywahls.com/tedxiowacity-minding-your-mitochondria-with-dr-terry-wahls; Wahls, T. with Adamson, E., *The Wahls Protocol: A Radical New Way to Treat All Chronic Autoimmune Conditions Using Paleo Principles*, Penguin: New York, 2014.

16. Jacka, F.N., O'Neil, A., Opie, R., et al., 'A randomised controlled trial of dietary improvement for adults with major depression (the 'SMILES' trial)', *BMC Med*, 2017, 15(1): 23.

17. Jacka, F.N., Pasco, J.A., Williams, L.J., 'Red meat consumption and mood and anxiety disorders', *Psychother Psychosom*, 2012, 81(3): 196–8.

Your Toolkit

How to Measure Body Fat

1. Swainson, M.G., Batterham, A.M., Tsakirides, C., et al., 'Prediction of whole-body fat percentage and visceral adipose tissue mass from five anthropometric variables', *PLOS ONE*, 2017, 12(5): e0177175.

What Blood Tests Should I Have?

1. Ridker, P.M., 'A test in context high-sensitivity c-reactive protein', *J Am Coll Cardiol*, 2016, 67(6): 712–723.

Index